Christine Eiser   J. Richard Eiser

Drug Education in Schools

An Evaluation of the "Double Take" Video Package

Springer-Verlag
New York Berlin Heidelberg
London Paris Tokyo

Christine Eiser
J. Richard Eiser
Department of Psychology
Washington Singer Laboratories
University of Exeter
Exeter EX4 4QG
England

With 10 Illustrations

Library of Congress Cataloging-in-Publication Data
Eiser, Christine.
Drug education in schools.
(Recent research in psychology)
Bibliography: p.
1. Teenagers—Great Britain—Drug use. 2. Drug abuse—Great Britain—Prevention. 3. Drug abuse—Study and teaching—Great Britain. 4. Video tapes in education. 5. Teenagers—Great Britain—Attitudes.
I. Eiser, J. Richard. II. Title. III. Series.
HV5824.Y68E37 1988 362.2'9 88-15957

This publication is based on research funded by the Department of Health and Social Security. However, the views expressed are those of the authors and not necessarily those of the DHSS.

Camera-ready copy provided by the authors.
Printed and bound by Edwards Brothers, Inc., Ann Arbor, Michigan.
Printed in the United States of America.

9 8 7 6 5 4 3 2 1

ISBN 0-387-96792-3 Springer-Verlag New York Berlin Heidelberg
ISBN 3-540-96792-3 Springer-Verlag Berlin Heidelberg New York

Recent Research in Psychology

PREFACE

"Double Take" is a drug education package, produced by the Department of Health and Social Security (DHSS) in conjunction with the Teachers' Advisory Council for Drug Education (TACADE) and the Institute for the Study of Drug Dependence (ISDD). The package was distributed at no cost to all secondary schools catering for pupils from 11 years and older in England and Wales during 1986. This research report is concerned with an evaluation of the package, particularly in terms of its acceptability to teachers and pupils.

"Double Take" is aimed primarily at pupils between 12 and 15 years of age. It consists of two videos, each with teachers' notes and pupils' exercises. The first, "Minder - A Little Bit of Give and Take", is based on a popular television series, and involved the main characters from the professional acting cast. It is produced in three parts, each of approximately 10 minutes in length. The video is less concerned with communicating 'facts' about drugs and more with imparting attitudes and skills necessary to deal with situations where drugs may be offered or available. It is therefore focused on coping skills and dealing with social pressures to take drugs. Above all, though, it comes across as a piece of television drama with an involving story-line, rather than as an 'educational' programme designed specifically for teaching purposes.

In the first part of the "Minder" video, the main characters are introduced. Shaun is a teenager from the North of England, who comes to London because his father is in prison. He contacts Arthur, an old friend of his father's, for help and somewhere to stay. Arthur is a businessman prone to deals of dubious legality, who is about to set off for a holiday on the Costa Brava. He therefore gives the job of looking after Shaun to his friend and "minder" Terry, an ex-boxer.

Shaun also contacts his cousin Tim, who is very unfriendly. Since his own parents are away, Tim plans a party, and Shaun is invited by Tim's girlfriend Sharon. In the second part of the video, Shaun goes to the party, and is confronted with a number of situations involving both legal and especially illegal drug-use. Shaun is offered heroin but refuses. After the party he decides to have nothing more to do with his cousin.

In the third part of the video, Arthur returns from holiday and attempts to sell some antique vases. Shaun recognizes these as belonging to Tim's parents. It becomes clear that Tim is stealing from his parents in order to pay for his heroin.

The rationale behind the teachers' notes and pupils' exercises is that "drug education is as much about people as it is about drugs". A course of five sessions, each approximately one hour in length, is recommended. Many of the exercises in the first session encourage pupils to consider the attitudes and behaviour of the main characters. In the second session, pupils consider the costs and benefits of drugs, and extent to which individuals are responsible for their own drug-taking behaviour. The third session is more focused on peer influence and how it operates. Pupils are encouraged to identify the skills necessary to deal with peer influence, and practice ways of saying "No". The fourth session is devoted to discussions about the stereotypes of drug-takers, and causes of drug-taking and possible ways of tackling the problem. It is suggested that the final session take the form of an overview of previous sessions, or alternative activities are recommended. These include talks from outside speakers (police, counsellors, social workers), collecting an anthology of poems about drugs, or mounting an exhibition for the rest of the school.

The second video, "Thinking Twice", is made in four parts, each of approximately 5 minutes in length. It is recommended that the video be shown as part of four separate sessions, each of at least 40 minutes duration. "Thinking Twice" takes the form of a theatre workshop in which young actors play out roles and comment on decisions about drugs which all young people encounter. The action takes place in three separate situations - a school visit to an imaginary museum in which both legal and illegal drugs are on display; a party; and at school. The main theme of the video is "to take things that are relatively familiar - such as coffee, alcohol, cigarettes - and to use them to demonstrate important principles also applicable to the less familiar, illegal drugs".

The first session focuses on the issues of defining drugs and distinguishing between the legal and illegal. Some basic information is also presented. The second session is more concerned with how drugs work, and the influence of dose, mood and situation on a drug's effectiveness. In the third session, pupils are encouraged to think about situations in which they might be offered legal or illegal drugs. Finally, it is suggested that bad habits in terms of drug-taking develop over a period of time, and pupils are encouraged to consider their own drug-taking behaviour and attitudes.

Neither video is intended to be the only approach to drug education that is adopted by a school. It is emphasized that drug-taking can occur for a number of reasons, and teachers are encouraged to be aware of, and integrate, other materials within their courses.

In addition to the free distribution of this package by the DHSS, the Department of Education and Science allocated £ 2 million in 1986 to be shared between the 96 Local Education Authorities for tackling drug abuse. This was sufficient to allow each Local Authority to appoint a full-time member of staff to stimulate and coordinate educational activities within the Authority. These Drugs Advisory Teachers were to advise teachers as to the availability of materials and to help them develop drug education curricula. They also arranged for teachers to attend training courses, so as to enable them to become familiar with a variety of approaches.

There have been a fair number of previous evaluations of drug education packages in schools. Many of these have been conducted in North America and have involved collaboration between the researchers and a limited number of schools or school authorities. Often the programmes are implemented by teachers who are specially trained for this purpose, rather than by those already employed in the schools concerned. Furthermore, the implementation of these programmes typically involves the commitment of many hours of curriculum time during the period of the trial. Such evaluation strategies essentially take the form of social psychological experiments conducted in the classroom rather than the laboratory, and follow much of the logic of classic experimental design in aiming for strong manipulations that have a maximal chance of success. The results of such research tell us whether programmes can be effective under optimal conditions. They may tell us rather less, however, about the effects one might expect when programmes are implemented by non-specialist teachers under the constraints of a general school system where every new form of educational input must compete for its share of curriculum time.

The evaluation to be reported was conducted deliberately within the context of such organizational restrictions. Our concern was less with the potential effectiveness of "Double Take" under optimal conditions. Rather, we were interested in the ways in which teachers themselves chose to adopt and integrate the package within existing courses and with the reactions of pupils in their schools. For this reason, many of the analyses are necessarily correlational, although we sought to introduce quasi-experimental comparisons where possible.

We acknowledge with gratitude the help we have received from many people at different stages of the research. Martin Böcker, Stephen Claxton-Oldfield, Kerstin Keil, Rachel Kirby, Sharon Lapham and Mary Pritchard helped with the collection and analysis of the data to be reported. Angela Boobyer, Joan FitzHenry, Sandy Salisbury and Kerstin Keil helped in the preparation of the manuscript. Margaret Draper, the Drugs Advisory Teacher for Devon, facilitated our collaboration with local schools. The many teachers and pupils who participated in the research itself deserve our special thanks.

Last but not least, we are grateful to the DHSS for their support, as well as for their encouragement at all stages of the project. The conclusions and views here expressed, though, are those of the authors and not necessarily those of the Department of Health and Social Security.

TABLE OF CONTENTS

1

Previous research on drug abuse and its prevention among school children

Difficulties in assessing the prevalence of drug abuse among school children

'Drug misuse' is generally taken to involve both (i) the non-medical use of drugs which are intended to be used as part of a prescribed course of medical treatment and (ii) the illicit use of drugs which have no accepted medical function (Home Office Report, 1986). Although it is not possible to measure the extent of drug-taking with a high degree of accuracy, much evidence is taken to suggest that drug misuse among young people in Britain has increased in recent years. Reports in both Britain (Home Office Report, 1986) and the United States (MacDonald, 1987) suggest that drug-taking increased dramatically during the 1960's, levelled off in the mid-1970's, and then began to increase again.

Estimates of the numbers involved in drug-misuse are based on several indirect indices. In Britain, one such indicator is the number of addicts who are formally notified to the Home Office by doctors. There was an approximate 25% increase in numbers notified between 1983 and 1984, and a similar number again between 1984 and 1985. Yet it is well-known that only a small proportion of the total number of addicts in the country are notified in this way (DHSS Report, 1982).

A second indicator refers to the numbers of seizures of drugs made by Customs Officers at ports and airports. Again, the number of seizures has increased substantially in recent years. Although the majority of seizures have involved cannabis, the number and quantity of heroin seizures is also increasing.

A third indicator involves the number of people dealt with for drug offences. Again, there have been substantial rises in the number of people found guilty of, or cautioned for, unlawful possession or trafficking in illegal drugs.

Other evidence has been accrued from a variety of sources: the police, counselling agencies, drug-dependency clinics and accident and emergency departments. Taken together, there is evidence that drug misuse among young people in Britain is increasing, and pervades all parts of the country.

In estimating prevalence rates among school-children, investigators have tended to rely on self-report measures. These measures are notoriously difficult to interpret, yet remain the only practical means of assessing prevalence of illicit drug use. Even where confidentiality is assured, different self-report measures may produce different results. Horan *et al.* (1974) found that 18% of their sample admitted to using drugs 'harder' than marijuana or hashish when interviewed, while 46% of an equivalent group admitted to this behaviour when responding to anonymous questionnaires. Inclusion of 'fake' drugs can give some indication of subjects who make extravagant drug-taking claims (Horan, 1972) but cannot wholly solve the problem.

An alternative approach which may act as an indirect indicator of drug-abuse has been suggested by Petchers and Singer (1987). They developed a self-administered 'perceived-benefit-of- drinking' scale. The instrument is designed to assess pupils' reasons for drinking alcohol. Five statements are each rated either 'true' or 'false'. The statements are shown in Table 1.1.

Pupils' responses were compared with self-reports of drinking behaviour. Those who saw there to be several advantages to drinking (i.e. rated more statements as 'true') were more likely to have been in trouble related to drinking, and to report being drunk in the previous 2 months. Petchers and Singer concluded that this simple questionnaire could be used as a preliminary indicator of problem drinking among adolescents, and suggest further that similar scales could be developed to aid in the detection of illicit drug-abuse. Unless a reliable physiological indicator of drug-abuse can be developed that is also practicable to administer on a large scale, measures such as these, despite their limitations, remain the primary methods available to estimate prevalence of substance abuse.

TABLE 1.1

Perceived Benefit-of-Drinking Scale

Circle either T (true) or F (false) for every sentence below

T F Drinking helps me forget any problems.

T F Drinking helps me be friendly.

T F Drinking helps me feel good about myself.

T F Drinking helps me relax.

T F Drinking helps me be friends with others who drink.

From Petchers & Singer (1987)

Prevalence of drug abuse among American and British school children

"Experimentation with cigarettes, alcohol, and marijuana appears to be the norm. Nearly 60% of all high school students will have smoked at least one marijuana cigarette prior to graduation, and similar contact with alcohol and tobacco is almost universal. Conspicuous minorities of the high school population have experimented with hallucinogens (14%), cocaine (13%), inhalents (12%), amphetamines (23%), and sedatives and tranquillizers (16%). ... about 10% of high school students have had contact with any form of opioids, and only 1.6% have specifically tried heroin." (Horan & Harrison, 1981, p.291)

These data, based on surveys by the U.S. Surgeon General (USPHS, 1979) and Johnston *et al.* (1979) suggest that a relatively high percentage of American youth experiment with illicit drugs while they are at school. The figures may overestimate the real extent of the problem, however, since they are based on pupils' reporting just one instance. The figures decline dramatically if use is defined as 'once or twice a month'. In this case, the prevalence of amphetamine misuse is 2.4% and less than 1% for all other drugs.

Surveys of British youth have been reviewed by Parker *et al.* (1986). Work in London, (Wiener, 1970) and Leeds (Hindmarch, 1972) suggested that approximately 10% of pupils claimed to have ever used a controlled drug, usually cannabis or amphetamine. Swift *et al.* (1974) surveyed pupils in schools in the north, south and midlands of England and reported similar prevalence rates. In the study by Swift *et al.* (1974), 4% of pupils admitted to regular use of illicit drugs. The surveys indicated that boys used drugs more than girls and that regular users were approximately 1 in 5 or 1 in 4 of all those who used drugs.

Wright and Pearl (1981) surveyed three comprehensive schools in Wolverhampton over an 11-year period, focussing on knowledge of drugs and whether or not pupils claimed to have ever been offered drugs. The proportion who had been offered drugs increased from 5% in 1969 to 10% in 1974 and 1979. Over the same period, cannabis replaced amphetamines as the drug most usually used.

A survey in Bristol (Parker *et al.*, 1986) involved pupils from four comprehensives. In all 890 4th formers (14-15 years) and 132 6th formers (17-18 years) completed questionnaires about their knowledge of drugs and people who took them. Fourth formers appeared knowledgeable about the names of illicit drugs, but were less informed about how such drugs were taken or of their effects and potential dangers. With the exception of cannabis, the most commonly mentioned drugs were also those least available - a finding that Parker *et al.* take as evidence that the pupils' knowledge is derived from adult sources rather than personal experience. In the Bristol survey, there was evidence that girls were as involved in drug abuse as boys, and the drugs most commonly abused were cannabis, hallucinogens and amphetamine. Fourth formers were more knowledgeable about the effects and dangers of solvent abuse than they were about the dangers of other illicit drugs. Approximately 20% of 4th formers claimed to have used solvents at some time. 28% of 4th formers and 61% of 6th formers had been offered drugs - at parties (35%), friends' houses (30%), in the street (30%), pubs or clubs (26%), school (21%), or elsewhere (17%). In comparison with the Wolverhampton survey (Wright & Pearl, 1981), the Bristol results suggest that drugs were more available and that more pupils are involved.

Patterns of drug abuse

Health education directed at preventing drug abuse is particularly important given suggestions that patterns of drug abuse follow a systematic progression. In the United States, Yamaguchi and Kandel (1984) followed a group of 16-year-olds over a nine year period. They describe a sequence of drug use from legal drugs (cigarettes or alcohol) to marijuana and other illegal drugs. Some differences in the pattern were noted for men and women, particularly that cigarettes are more important for women than men in determining the course of illicit drug use. In a subsequent paper (Kandel & Yamaguchi, 1984) they argued that the major risk for initiation into cigarettes, alcohol and marijuana abuse is over by 20 years, and to illicit drugs other than cocaine by 21 years. Those who have not experimented with these drugs by 21 years are unlikely to ever do so. Initiation into prescribed psychoactive drugs occurs at a later age and continues up to 25 years or so. The use of marijuana declines from approximately 25 years.

Assessing the outcome of drug education

Against this background, there has been a recognition of the need to educate young people about the dangers of drug abuse. Drug prevention programmes have not, however, always met with approval. There have been substantial fears that education of this kind will result in more permissive attitudes to drug-taking and increased incidences of experimentation. Objections that are often voiced against drug education have been summarized by Stuart (1974).

Drug education ... "might exacerbate drug use by (a) providing students with sufficient information to facilitate the initiation of use; (b) providing students with facts that overcome the prejudices that had been inhibiting use; (c) desensitizing the students about drugs through repeated discussion of drug concepts ...; (d) leading students to think of themselves as potential drug users ...; (e) changing attitudes that were the bastion of defense against drug use; or (f) occasionally including inaccurate or biased information, which undermines the credibility of the basic educational message." (Stuart, 1974, p.190).

Despite such reservations, various drug education programmes have been developed. The aims of these programmes are typically threefold:- (a) to increase knowledge about drugs; (b) to promote healthy attitudes towards the use of drugs and (c) to decrease potential drug abuse behaviour.

In practice, objections can be made to all three approaches.

(a) *Knowledge gain*

One of the most basic objections to this approach centres on the claim that increasing drug knowledge can lead to more favourable attitudes towards drugs (Stuart & Schuman, 1972; Swisher & Horan, 1973; Swisher, Crawford, Goldstein & Yura, 1971). Smart and Fejer (1974) argued that some pupils who had decided not to take drugs did so following intervention programmes. Their fears were allayed by the drug education programmes and they became more willing to experiment. In a related study (Stuart, 1974), it was further claimed that increases in drug knowledge resulted in greater drug abuse behaviour. In fact, the increases in drug abuse behaviour were very small. "For example, on a 1-5 scale where 1 was defined as 'no use' and 2 as 'once or twice per year', experimental seventh graders changed in marijuana consumption from a pretest mean of 1.11 to a post-test mean of 1.24, in contrast to the control group where the mean rose from 1.05 to 1.12", (Horan & Harrison, 1981).

In their enthusiastic attempts to educate people about the dangers of drug abuse, educators have, on occasion, blatantly miseducated them through exaggerating and distorting some of the facts about drugs. Halleck (1970, p.2), for example, summarizes the approach often adopted in early prevention programmes:-

"The most prevalent but least effective theme in the drug education program is to 'scare the hell out of them'. Too often the program consists of one or more meetings at which a local physician, a law enforcement officer, and perhaps a former addict will endlessly catalogue the horrible consequences of drug usage. The physician will stress the degree to which drugs can produce bodily damage. The law enforcement officer will gravely talk about the increasing flow of drugs into the community and will throw in a few anecdotes about young people he has seen ruined by drugs. Sometimes he will even bring in displays of confiscated drugs to show his presumably horrified audience. The former addict, who is usually the star performer, will recount his sordid experiences as a drug user and will glowingly report the salutatory effects of his reformation. It is an interesting show which has much of the flavor of an old-fashioned revival meeting."

The result is that pupils may well feel that more accurate information about drugs can be obtained from drug users than from orthodox classroom teaching.

The third problem with using knowledge gain as an indicator of success of a prevention programme is that researchers differ widely in their ideas about what constitutes drug knowledge. It may well be academic, cutting across such diverse disciplines as biology, chemistry and the law; it may be 'street-wise'. Previous research looking at changes in knowledge as a function of prevention has not always been clear about the type of knowledge being assessed.

(b) *Attitude change*

In some studies, attitude scales have been devised and used to assess the effectiveness of intervention programmes. The assumption is that if negative attitudes towards drugs can be demonstrated, then the programme has achieved a degree of success. Horan and Harrison (1981) have argued that there is a lack of consensus among researchers about the items that should constitute such a drugs scale. In particular, they point to two errors frequently made in developing these scales. The first is that drug attitudes may be confounded with misinformation. The statement, "The use of marijuana inevitably leads to the use of heroin", is one example. Agreement with such a statement may indicate a negative attitude toward drugs; it may also indicate that the respondent, quite mistakenly, believes it to be true. The second error involves the confounding of drug attitudes with politics. For example, the statement "Some drug laws are too harsh" is open to a variety of interpretations, given the fact that there is little consensus of opinion as to the appropriate punishment for drug offenders. Indeed, there is wide variability in the severity of punishment for a given drug offence across countries, or even within the United States.

(c) *Behaviour change*

Ultimately, the goal of drug education programmes is to reduce the probability that young people will begin to take drugs, or at least progress from experimental to habitual use. Longitudinal evaluations of such behavioural outcomes however, are rare. More typically, finances are not available, researchers do not have the staying power, and a host of intervening factors can occur between the programme and the onset of drug-taking behaviour that make simple cause-effect conclusions impossible. In order to assess behaviour change, therefore, researchers are forced to ask subjects to estimate their consumption of various drugs, and look for changes after the intervention programme. Such self-report measures as discussed previously are, of course, open to bias.

Theoretical bases of prevention programmes

Early work in the drug prevention field centred almost exclusively on an *information-based* approach. According to decision-theory (Bauman, 1980), the choice between two or more alternatives, (e.g. experimenting with or abstaining from drugs) is dependent on the perceived utilities of each alternative and their probabilities of occurrence. It follows that by providing information about the dangers of drug abuse and suggesting the high probability of adverse consequences, young people will be deterred from drug abuse behaviour. Indirect support for this model was provided by Halliday (1976) who showed that drug attitudes could be manipulated by varying the kind of information given. A large number of studies, in fact, have shown that drug education programmes devised to increase knowledge about drugs are relatively successful (for a review see Horan & Harrison 1981), i.e. in terms of increasing knowledge. However, that is all that they tend to achieve. There is little evidence that increased knowledge about drugs has a systematic effect on attitude or behaviour.

(a) *Information based approaches*

The information-based approach has been widely criticized (Leventhal & Cleary, 1980; Leventhal, Safer & Panagis, 1983). In particular, the inaccurate information that is often given regarding the negative consequences of drug abuse is at variance with the initial experiences and testimony of friends. In addition, there is rarely any acknowledgement of the perceived positive effects of drug use (in the opinion of many young people, taking drugs can be fun or exciting or help relieve negative moods). Horan and Harrison (1981, p. 320) note that there is little likelihood of an information-based approach changing attitudes or behaviour until 'its implementation corresponds to the decision-making framework on which it ought to be based'.

(b) *Induced cognitive dissonance*

A limited number of drug education programmes have been based on Cognitive Dissonance Theory (Festinger, 1957). The main assumption of this theory is that individuals are motivated to seek consistency between their thoughts, emotions and motor behaviours. By exposing individuals to information which makes them aware of states of inconsistency that exist within their own value-attitude system, it is expected that attitude change will result. Swisher and Horan (1972) categorized subjects according to whether they preferred direct experiences (e.g. playing football), or indirect experiences (e.g. watching football). Subjects were told which category they belonged to, and were then exposed to the argument that since drugs were another way to mediate experience, then the value preference for direct experience was inconsistent with holding a prodrug attitude. As hypothesized, those who preferred direct experiences shifted their attitudes in a conservative direction.

Attempts to replicate this study have not been successful (Warner, Swisher & Horan, 1973). It is difficult, too, to see how different this approach really is from an information-based approach.

(c) *Group counselling*

The approach, based on principles of modelling and classical or operant conditioning, has also achieved only limited success. The approach capitalizes on the observation that there are a variety of alternatives to taking drugs, all of which can produce similar positive consequences. The rationale is that the group leader ignores any prodrug attitudes expressed by members of the group, but attempts to foster antidrug attitudes by cueing and selective reinforcement. Using this technique, Warner, Swisher and Horan (1973) reported that drug attitudes changed in a conservative direction.

(d) *Decision-making and problem-solving: The 'life-skills' approach*

The new phase in drug education began in the 1970's, in response to a heightened awareness about *why* individuals take drugs. Research increasingly suggested that individuals who take drugs differ from others on a number of dimensions. Drug-users are more likely to do badly in school, to engage in anti-social behaviour (such as lying or stealing, Jessor *et al* 1971). They are variously described as lacking in self-confidence, self-esteem, self-satisfaction and assertiveness, while at the same time being rebellious, impulsive and impatient to assume adult roles. Social skills approaches to drug education have been developed to increase self-esteem and interpersonal skills and encourage participation in alternative activities.

'Social skills' are primarily communicative in function (Swisher, 1976) and refer to the "ability to cope with interpersonal relationships" (Argyris, 1968). There is evidence that a range of social skills are acquired during adolescence, particularly those involving assertiveness, expression of opinion, ability to disagree and refuse, make requests and initiate conversations (Pentz, 1980; Schinke, 1981). The corollary of this research is that adolescents who fail to develop these social skills are more likely to develop anti-social behaviours, such as delinquency, truancy, agression and academic and social withdrawal (Goldstein *et al.*, 1978).

Acknowledging that there may be a relation between the failure to develop social skills and anti-social behaviour including drug-taking, has resulted in drug education programmes which attempt to improve mastery of basic social skills. "Social skills training" involves "mutual benefit and maintenance of personal integrity" (Schinke, 1981). The techniques used include modelling, rehearsal, feedback with social reinforcement and extended practice. These techniques may be used singly or in combination, and focus on developing both the cognitive and behavioural aspects of any particular skill.

The approach was pioneered by Evans (1981) as the basis of school-based anti-smoking campaigns. His basic assumption was that individuals begin to smoke because of peer pressure and an accompanying inability to resist these influences and 'say no' to drugs. The assumption in itself has subsequently been shown to be an over-simplification. While there is undoubtedly a high correlation between an individual's substance use and that of friends, it is debatable whether these associations are the result of peer pressure or represent a process of mutual self-selection. A related objection centres on the fact that, since most adolescents do not smoke or take illegal drugs, peer pressure should operate to reduce, rather than increase, the frequency of these behaviours. Certainly, empirical evidence does not support the view that adolescent drug-use is the inevitable result of peer pressure. Kandel (1978) found that friendship pairs were usually congruent (85%) with regard to marijuana use. Where friendship pairs were initially incongruent, either marijuana use did not change (44%), or both members became non-users (34%). Only in 17% of pairs did the original non-user subsequently take marijuana. Thus, selection of friends may be a more critical determinant of drug-use than any effects of conformity pressure.

The 'life-skills' approach

The more recent extension of social skills theory assumes that individuals take drugs because they lack appropriate social and decision-making skills. Programmes have varied in the extent to which they focus on promoting life-skills necessary to cope with drug-related situations, (Flay, 1985). This is described as the *social inoculation* approach (Maguire, 1964). A related approach *life-skills training* includes attempts to teach pupils skills appropriate to a variety of situations, not only those related to drugs (Botvin, 1983).

"Some of the general cognitive-behavioural techniques incorporated into the LST (Life-Skills Training) program include cognitive strategies for enhancing self-esteem (e.g. goal-setting, behaviour change techniques, replacing negative self-statements with positive ones); techniques for resisting persuasive (advertising) appeals (e.g., identifying persuasive appeals, formulating counter-arguments); cognitive-behavioural self-management techniques for coping with anxiety (e.g. relaxation training, mental rehearsal); verbal and non-verbal communications skills; and a variety of social skills (e.g. initiating social interactions, conversational skills, heterosexual ("dating") skills, complimenting, verbal and nonverbal assertive skills). These skills are taught using a combination of instruction, modelling, rehearsal, feedback and reinforcement, and extended practice through homework assignments". (Botvin, 1983, p.129)

Evaluations of 'life-skills' approaches

Positive effects of education programmes based on social skills approaches to preventing smoking have been reported (Arkin *et al.*, 1981;

Botvin, 1983; Evans *et al.*, 1981; Flay *et al.*, 1983; Hurd *et al.*, 1980; McAlister *et al.*, 1980; Perry *et al.*, 1980). There are claims that smoking can be prevented or delayed for up to 3 years following these programmes (Luepker *et al.*, 1983). In addition, there is a reduction of 50% in the initiation of smoking behaviour (Evans *et al.*, 1979; Perry, Maccoby & McAlister, 1980).

Other researchers have not, however, found any positive effects of related programmes (Blum *et al.*, 1978; Schaps *et al.*, 1984), while others have found that the effects dissipate quickly, and 'booster' sessions are required.

There have been fewer evaluations of broad-based life-skills approaches aimed at improving social skills generally rather than restricted to those involved in smoking or other drug-related behaviours. Exceptions are a series of reports by Botvin and colleagues.

Botvin (1983) used the life-skills approach to teach 1200 pupils drawn from 10 schools. All pupils were from white, predominantly middle-class families. The programme was extensive (at least in comparison to British interventions)involving life-skills teaching once a week for 15 weeks. During the first year following the programme, there appeared to be substantial effects on tobacco, alcohol and marijuana use. The programme appeared to be associated with a 71% reduction in total marijuana use and 83% reduction in regular (weekly or daily) marijuana use.

Objections and criticisms of social skills approaches

Early reports claiming 50% reductions in smoking behaviour as a result of social skills programmes were probably exaggerated. Most evaluations have been conducted soon after the intervention programme. In fact, habitual cigarette use only becomes established among older pupils. There is as yet, no evidence that social skills programmes reduce habitual cigarette smoking.

There have been many other criticisms made of the methods used to evaluate these programmes. Battjes & Bell (1985) list some of these as follows:-

(a) Attrition is a problem in any long-term evaluation. There is some evidence that pupils who are lost to intervention programmes represent a disproportionately high number of those likely to use tobacco and other substances. Particularly if attrition rates differ across conditions, an apparent treatment effect may be an artifact of loss of high risk pupils from a treatment group.

(b) There has been little acknowledgement of the possibility of Hawthorne effects. Comparison groups should be included who receive programmes similar to the social skills packages but without the specific elements thought to be essential.

(c) More attention also needs to be paid to the specific components of the programmes that are responsible for promoting changes in behaviour.

(d) Programme evaluations have generally been based in white, middle-class schools, and it is not clear as to how generalizable they may be, especially for groups from deprived, or ethnic backgrounds.

(e) There is little acknowledgement of individual variation in how the programme is received. The social skills approach assumes that individuals take drugs as a result of social influences. Yet other reasons may well be implicated, including poor home background or academic failure. Those who are at most risk in terms of drug use appear to use drugs for reasons other than social influences (Robins & Przybeck, 1985).

(f) Some evaluations have focused on the impact of the programme on those who have never smoked; others in terms of their impact on regular smokers. In fact, programmes need to be acceptable to all pupils, regardless of individual variation in substance use, since there is no possibility within a school setting of targetting education at particular sub-groups.

(g) Many programmes use highly skilled and motivated teachers. It is not clear how easily the programmes can be implemented by the majority of teachers. Moskowitz *et al.* (1982) showed there to be considerable variation in how programmes were implemented, even among teachers who had received in-service training.

Comparing formal 'information-giving' teaching styles with less formal discussion groups

It has been suggested that the mode of presentation may be the most important variable in determining the effectiveness of any drug education programme (Kinsey *et al.*, 1975; Bruhn *et al.*, 1975; Mathews, 1975). In fact, there is little systematic research to compare the differential effectiveness of drugs programmes which adopt a 'formal' information-giving approach with those which adopt an effective group discussion approach or those which focus on videos. The issue is one which is also central in other areas of health education. Peterson and Ridley-Johnson (1984), for example, attempted to prepare well children in the classroom for emergency hospital admission by means of a formal lecture or film. Both methods succeeded in reducing children's hospital-related fears, but only the film resulted in any increase in knowledge of hospital procedures and equipment.

Few studies have investigated the impact of different teaching styles on the success of drug education programmes. Smith (1973) divided college students into three groups; 1) a traditional, teacher-centred, information-giving approach, 2) a group-centred, affective approach and 3) a control group which took part in a discussion of non-drug related problems. Only those experiencing the group-centred approach showed significant attitude changes in the desired direction. A similar procedure was adopted by Morgan and Hayward (1976). Subjects experienced either a formal lecture series with little discussion allowed, or more informal discussion groups. Unfortunately, there were no changes in attitude among those experiencing the group-centred approach. However, there were some indications of shifts toward permissive attitudes to drugs among those in the formal lecture group.

In a third study, Stuart (1974) allocated 13- and 15-year olds to one of three teaching groups. Both the content and teaching style of the groups was varied. The content of the course focused on 1) 'milder' drugs (e.g. marijuana, nicotine); 2) 'harder' drugs (heroin, hallucinogens) or 3) a combination of both of these. The style of teaching was varied between formal teacher-led instructions or discussion groups. For all subjects, data on past and present drug use, attitudes and knowledge were collected before and after the programme and at 4-month follow-up. In addition, a control group received no drug education at all.

The results can only be described as disappointing. There were no differences between the two experimental groups in attitude and knowledge. However, immediately after the programme and at 4-month follow-up there were differences between experimental and control group subjects. Experimental subjects were more knowledgeable, reported greater alcohol, marijuana and LSD use and were more likely to be marijuana sellers than controls.

To date, then, there is little systematic evidence to suggest that informal approaches to drug education generally have greater potential than more traditional approaches.

However, Botvin (1983) has presented some evidence that life-skills approaches to drug prevention may be implemented more successfully by peer-leaders than by teachers.

Evaluations of the effectiveness of drug-education programmes

In summary, then there have been a large number of attempts to evaluate the effectiveness of smoking, alcohol and drug prevention programmes (for reviews see Janiver *et al.*, 1980; Kinder *et al.*, 1980; Schaps *et al.*, 1980, Schaps *et al.* 1981; Staulcup *et al.*, 1979). For the most part, the programmes appear to enjoy only limited success. There is commonly an increase in knowledge following these programmes, and occasionally minor changes in attitudes. However, neither knowledge nor attitude is clearly associated with drug-use, (Schegel & Norris, 1980; Maddox & McCall, 1964; Alexander & Campbell, 1968). The long-term effectiveness of these programmes in terms of preventing drug-abuse has not been established.

Despite this apparent failure, new methods of teaching pupils about drugs continue to be developed. If we are to assess the success of these programmes, it is clear that behavioural measures based on pupils' intentions to take drugs, or their subsequent drug-usage, are inadequate. Along with the development of new programmes, we need also to develop new insights into how to measure success.

Similar points have been made by Weisheit (1983), who argues that prevention programmes fulfil a need in curriculum development. He argues that alcohol and drug prevention programmes are generally regarded as 'unsuccessful' but so too, by comparative criteria, are delinquency prevention programmes (Hackler, 1978) and sex education (Smith & Gorry, 1980). Nevertheless, programmes are developed and are integrated into the curriculum. Whatever the scientific evidence as to the immediate efficacy of these programmes, there clearly is a body of public opinion that regards such primary prevention programmes as essential within the regular school-curriculum. For example, alcohol education is mandatory in most states of America (Milgram 1976). "The educational program is not only an effort to change adolescent drinking behaviour, but is just as importantly a symbolic act which signals concerned interest groups that some action is being taken to deal with the problem" (Weisheit, 1983, p.76).

In a field like drug education, evaluation of the effectiveness of any intervention is constrained by two main sets of difficulties: the fact that 'hard' data on effectiveness, such as reduction in morbidity, or in notified cases of drug abuse, may take many years to become apparent, and even then, any change may be difficult to attribute to a single intervention; and the fact that those who receive the intervention (and particularly those who make most thorough use of it) typically constitute a self-selected, and therefore non-random, sample.

Faced with these difficulties, researchers have often relied on 'softer' data, such as people's estimates of how likely an intervention is to work. Whereas such estimates are interesting for what they may reveal about the attitudes of the people concerned, no clear justification is usually provided for treating such guesses as valid predictors of effectiveness itself. In our view, it is therefore necessary to base the design of an evaluation on assumptions concerning the nature of the *process* that can connect the offer of information at one end with differences in acquired habits at the other. In other words, even where one cannot tell whether an intervention *has yet* worked, one can still attempt to find out how well it is satisfying certain conditions that may be assumed to be necessary for eventual effectiveness. Such an approach has the additional merit of pointing to possible areas of improvement, if such conditions are not fulfilled.

We consider that the necessary conditions for effectiveness of a package such as "Double Take" include the following two main sets of considerations. The first applies to the reactions of teachers and the second to that of pupils.

(a) *Teachers' reactions.* For the package to be effective at all, it must first of all be accepted by the schools. To be maximally effective, however, it cannot just be 'accepted', but must be used more widely and repetitively, must be integrated into the curriculum as an important rather than marginal element, and must be reinforced with follow-up discussions and activities of various kinds. We intend to assess how well these conditions have been met, and in particular, to attempt to identify factors that differentiate those schools which use the package more, rather than less, extensively and enthusiastically. Such factors may include not only 'demographic' or 'descriptive' variables (e.g. size of school, catchment area), but also organizational variables (e.g. Does the head teacher make the main decision on how extensively the package is to be used, or are other staff involved in the decision?), as well as the attitudes and beliefs concerning drugs and drug abuse held by the teachers concerned (e.g. Do they believe it to be a relevant problem for them? Why do they think young people take drugs? What do they think is the best form of discussion?).

(b) *Pupils' reactions.* Even if the package is used extensively, its effectiveness will be limited if pupils (and particularly those who may be most 'at risk') fail to attend to it, or understand it. Attention and comprehension will depend both on the activities of the teachers and on the content of the package itself. As regards content, there is a general question of how the irds content, there is a general question of how the information or message presented is going to be viewed in terms of pupils' existing attitudes and beliefs about drugs and drug abuse. It is important also that the information in the package not only is assimilated when first presented, but is retained for later use, notably in contexts where drugs are offered and need to be refused. Again, our assessment of pupils' reactions will attempt to go beyond mere indications of approval to determine how well such conditions are being met.

2

A survey of the extent of use of "Double Take" in schools and teachers' evaluations of the package

Introduction

This study was undertaken to find out how widely "Double Take" was being used in schools, and how well it had been received by teachers. To be effective at all, a first requirement must be that teachers adopt the package and implement it in a desirable fashion. This means that the package needs to be integrated as an important rather than a marginal element of the curriculum, used widely and repetitively and be reinforced with follow-up discussions and activities of various kinds. The aim of this first study was to assess how well these conditions had been met. In addition, we attempted to determine some of the factors that might affect how well the package was integrated within the curriculum. These included:

(1) information about the type of school, its size and whether or not the pupils came from deprived backgrounds.

(2) characteristics of teachers, in terms of personal variables including sex and subject taught, as well as their general attitudes to drug-taking. In particular, we assessed their attitudes to:

(1) why young people start to take drugs and

(2) how best to persuade people not to take drugs

Procedure and questionnaire

A list of all the schools who had placed an order for 'Double Take' was obtained from the distributors by the D.H.S.S. A random sample of those who had placed the order before the end of August 1986 were then contacted. (This was approximately 1 in 10 of the schools).

The questionnaire was sent by post to the individual schools who had placed the original order for "Double Take", with a covering note asking that it be passed to the person in school with most experience of its use. A reply-paid envelope was included for reply. The questionnaires were posted on 4th December 1986. A follow-up letter and another reply-paid envelope was sent to all non-respondents at the end of January 1987.

Teachers' Questionnaire

We first asked for the name and position in school of the individual completing the questionnaire, which was divided into the following sections.

Demographic information

Demographic information was collected about the school, noticeably the size (in terms of number of pupils); type (independent or maintained; selective or comprehensive, and sex of pupils); age-range; number of full-time teachers and teacher-pupil ratio. Teachers were also asked what percentage of pupils received free school meals (if appropriate) as a gross indicator of deprivation.

Process of decision-making before ordering "Double-Take"

Teachers were asked if there was still a copy of "Double Take" in the school, and whether the initial decision to order it was taken by (a) a staff meeting (b) memo or (c) individual discussions. We asked how many teachers had since seen the video. We also asked if parents had seen the video, and if the school had organized 'parent evenings' about drugs.

Drug education in the school

Teachers were asked to estimate the average number of curriculum hours during (a) 1985-6 and (b) 1986-7 devoted, or to be devoted, firstly to drug education in general and secondly to the use of "Double Take" (and the exercises based on it). This was done separately for each age group (11-12, 12-13, 13-14, 14-15, and 15-16 years). Teachers were also asked in which parts of the curriculum the video was used (spare periods, social education/tutor groups, health education, biology/science, English, other), and whether or not anyone from outside the school (medical staff, police, health education officers) were also involved on a regular basis.

There were then a series of questions to investigate the relative use of the separate parts of the video ("Minder" and "Thinking Twice") and the exercises based on them. Teachers were also asked to rate their personal opinion of the two parts and the accompanying exercises, and whether or not they had devised any exercises themselves.

We questionned whether or not other drug education programmes were used, and if so, why these were considered preferable to "Double Take". Teachers were also asked if they, or any other teacher at the school, had attended any TACADE (Teachers' Advisory Council for Drug Education) or LEA (Local Education Authority) drug advisory courses on drug education, and what the school policy was regarding pupils found experimenting with drugs.

Teachers' personal attitudes to drug taking

Teachers were asked to rate 20 statements (on a series of 7-point scales from definitely no to definitely yes) concerning why they believed 'young people start to take drugs like heroin'. They were then asked to rate a further 12 statements concerned with how best to persuade young people not to try drugs like heroin.

Finally, teachers were asked if they had any general comments about "Double Take" and if they would be prepared for us to involve some of the pupils in further research concerned with "Double Take". A copy of the questionnaire is shown in Appendix A.

Results

Perhaps because of the time of year, the teachers were generally slow to respond. 268 questionnaires were returned within 6 weeks. A further 207 were returned within 2 months of the reminder letter. The analysis therefore included 475 replies (47.5%). 40 were returned over an even longer period and were not included in the analyses. In addition, 47 letters were received explaining why teachers were unable to complete the questionnaire. Thus 56.2% of the sample communicated in some way.

Information about the teachers who completed the questionnaires

Sex. Of the 475 respondents, 123 (25.0%) were males, 210 (44.2%) were females and 142 (29.9%) did not answer this question.

Position in school. The largest group of respondents were head teachers (45.1%), followed by deputy head teachers (24.7%). Others included year-heads (4.7%), tutors (2.3%) and 'other' (20.2%). This information was not given by 15 (3.2%) of respondents.

Subject taught by respondent. Many of the respondents (42.3%) did not give this information, presumably reflecting the large number of non-teaching principals in the sample. The subjects taught by other respondents included biology (16.7%), home economics (3.9%), pastoral, social and moral education (PSME)(25.6%), health education (9.1%), religion (9.5%) and other including English (11.8%).

Attendance on drug education courses. Teachers were asked if they, or anyone else in the school, to their knowledge, had attended a course on drug education. 25.7% said that nobody in the school had attended any such course. Courses run by TACADE on drug education generally (11.1%) and "Double Take" specifically (2.5%) were mentioned by others. 23.4% had attended courses organised by Local Education Authority Drug Advisory Teachers. 20.2% of teachers had attended more than one course.

Information about the schools

Of the total sample, 16.0% of replies were from independent schools. 61.1% of schools were for both boys and girls, with 7.8% being for boys only and 9.9% for girls only. (Where frequencies do not add up to 100%, this is because teachers failed to complete all sections of the questionnaire). The age-range of pupils is shown in Figure 2.1; most schools catered for the 11-16 or 11-18 years range. The number of pupils ranged from less than 199 to more than 1800 and the distribution is shown in Figure 2.2. The number of full-time teachers is shown in Figure 2.3, with a range of less than 9 to more than 100. The pupil-teacher ratio varied from 9/1 to 35/1.

FIGURE 2.1

Age range of pupils

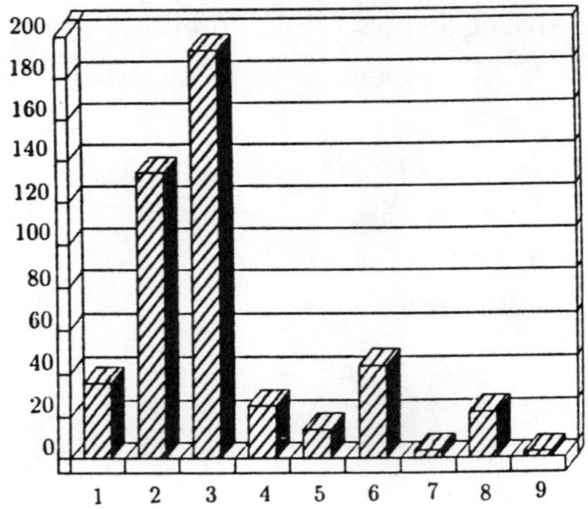

1 = 10 - 13 4 = 12 - 16 7 = 16 - 18
2 = 11 - 16 5 = 12 - 18 8 = other answer
3 = 11 - 18 6 = 13 - 18 9 = no answer

FIGURE 2.2

Number of pupils in school

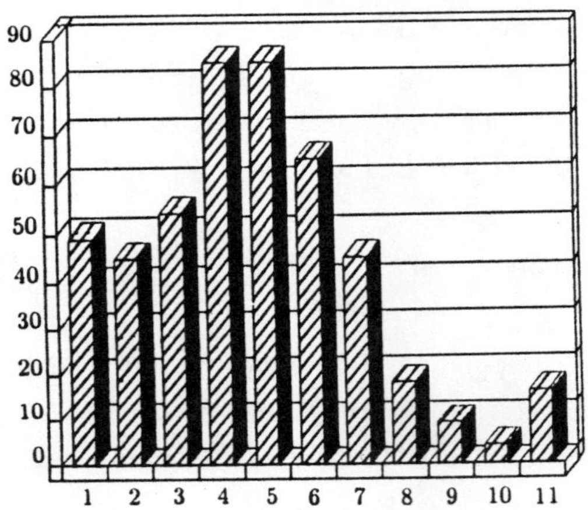

1 = 0 - 199 5 = 800 - 999 9 = 1600 - 1799
2 = 200 - 399 6 = 1000 - 1199 10 = more than 1800
3 = 400 - 599 7 = 1200 - 1399 11 = no answer
4 = 600 - 799 8 = 1400 - 1599

FIGURE 2.3

Number of teachers in school

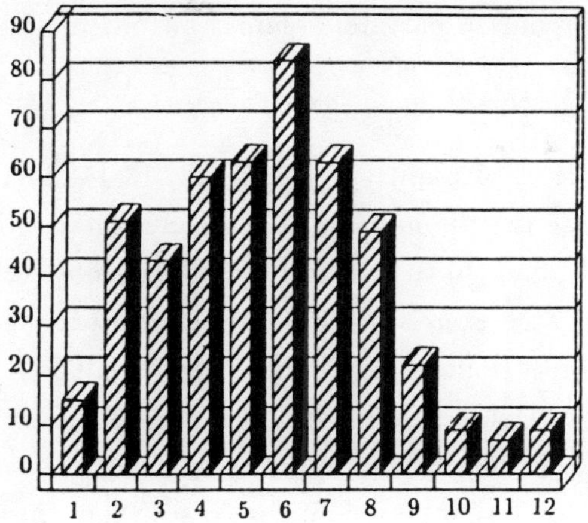

1 = 0 - 9	5 = 40 - 49	9 = 80 - 89
2 = 10 - 19	6 = 50 - 59	10 = 90 - 99
3 = 20 - 29	7 = 60 - 69	11 = more than 100
4 = 30 - 39	8 = 70 - 79	12 = no answer

How the decision to order "Double Take" was made

Of the 475 schools included in the analysis, all but 13 still had a copy available. (Among these 13, the video had either been lost, stolen, or taken by a teacher who was leaving to go to another school.) The decision to order "Double Take" was generally made by individual discussion between teachers (69.1%). In 10.5% of cases, decisions were taken by memo. Only for 2.1% of schools was the decision taken by a staff meeting. Other responses could not easily be categorized (7.4%) but included comments such as 'nobody remembers', or 'nobody ordered - it was just sent to us'. 11.0% of respondents did not answer this question.

The number of teachers involved in the decision was generally low. Only 1 or 2 teachers were involved in over half the schools (63.8%). Similarly, the number of teachers who had seen "Double Take" was low. In over half the schools, (51.4%), between 1 and 4 teachers had seen the video.

Involvement of parents

Few schools had given parents the opportunity to see the video, and almost half (44.6%) had not organized any parents' evenings about drugs.

A small proportion (12.0%) had organized one evening for parents, and a further 8.6% had organised more than one. The rest (33.5%) stated that they had not yet organized parents' evenings but intended to in the future.

The place of "Double Take" in the curriculum

For each age-level of pupils (11-12, 12-13, 13-14, 14-15, 15-16 years) we tried to estimate (a) the number of curriculum hours devoted to drug education generally, and (b) the number of hours devoted to "Double Take" including the associated exercises. Estimates were attempted for the school year 1985-86 (before "Double Take" was widely available) and the school year 1986-87 (when "Double Take" was more generally distributed). Figure 2.4 shows the number of curriculum hours devoted to drug education for each age-year over the 2 year period. It can be seen that the average number of hours is relatively stable, being lowest for the youngest pupils and peaking for 14-15 year old pupils. Figure 2.5 shows the number of schools using "Double Take" over the 2 years. "Double Take" is used more for all ages of pupils in the year 1986-87 compared with the previous year. Figure 2.6 shows the degree to which "Double Take" makes a contribution to drug education generally. For 13-14 year olds, on average, "Double Take" makes up half a course, and slightly more for years 14-15 and 15-16.

In many schools, "Double Take" is used as part of Social Education (61.2%) or Health Education (41.9%) courses. In other schools drugs are dealt with in biology (15.9%) or English (4.4%) courses. Only 17% of schools used "Double Take" to cover spare periods or staff absences. In 24.6% of schools, the package was used in more than one of these types of lesson and/or in some other part of the curriculum such as religious education. These data are shown in Figure 2.7.

On average, 3.34 (range = 1–25) teachers were involved in using "Double Take" in a school. Schools also involved a school nurse or doctor (8.9%), LEA Drugs Advisor (8.9%), or Health Education Officer (3.2%). 30.2% of schools involved more than one of these and/or other helpers (most frequently the police, but also priests and ex-drug addicts).

FIGURE 2.4

Number of schools using Drug Education (1985-86 and 1986-87)

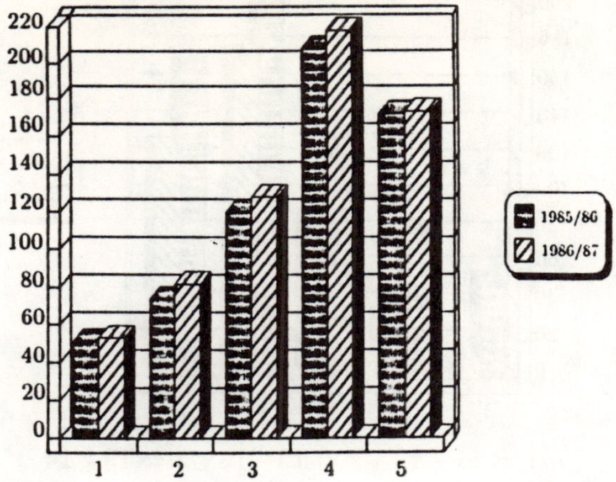

1 = 11 - 12   2 = 12 - 13   3 = 13 - 14
4 = 14 - 15   5 = 15 - 16   (Age groups)

FIGURE 2.5

Use of 'Double Take' (1985-86 and 1986-87)

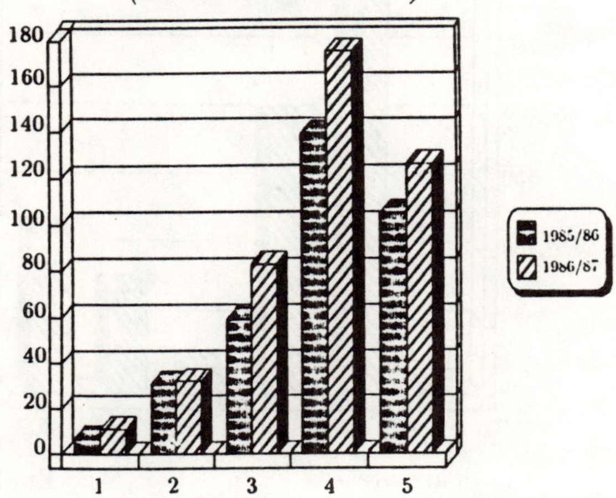

1 = 11 - 12   2 = 12 - 13   3 = 13 - 14
4 = 14 - 15   5 = 15 - 16   (Age groups)

FIGURE 2.6

Drug Education and the use of 'Double Take'

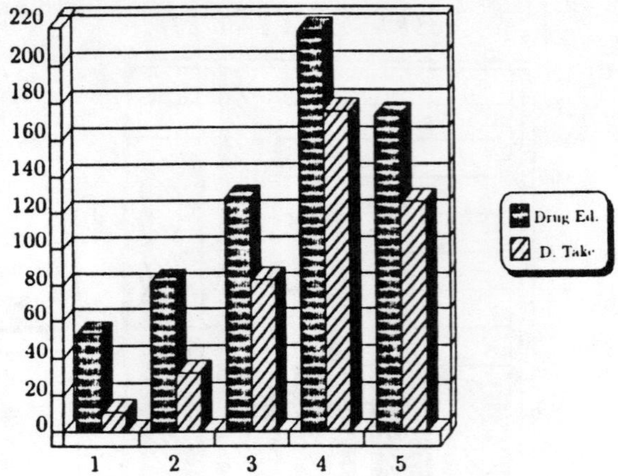

1 = 11 - 12   2 = 12 - 13   3 = 13 - 14
4 = 14 - 15   5 = 15 - 16   (Age groups)

FIGURE 2.7

Part of curriculum used for 'Double Take'

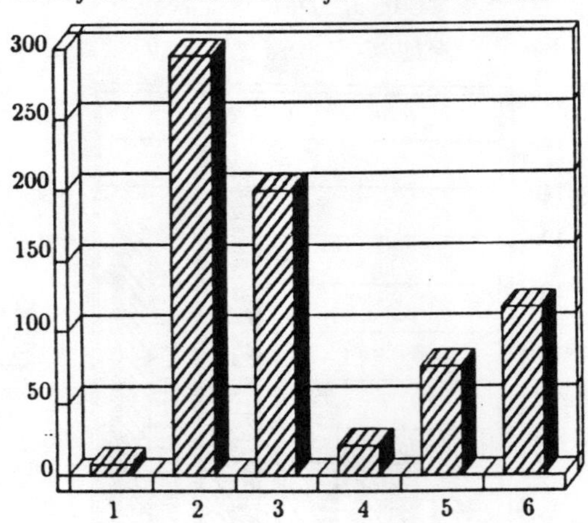

1 = Spare preiods
2 = Soc. Educ. - Tut. groups
3 = Health education
4 = English
5 = Biology
6 = other

How "Double Take" was used

Teachers were asked how much emphasis was placed on the two parts of "Double Take". Most teachers used both parts equally (35.9%) or placed much more emphasis on "Minder" (48.3%). Very few teachers placed emphasis on "Thinking Twice" (5.5%), though there was some difference between teachers within a school. Where teachers were using the video "Minder", they used the accompanying exercises 'selectively' (80.0%); 'closely' (7.1%) or 'not at all' (7.9%). Where teachers were using the "Thinking Twice" video, they used the accompanying exercises 'selectively' (71.9%), 'closely' (5.1%) or 'not at all' (23.1%).

Teachers' ratings of "Double Take"

Teachers were asked to rate the whole package, each video, and each set of exercises, separately on 7-point scales (from 'very unhelpful' to 'very helpful'). As shown in Figures 2.8, 2.9 and 2.10, teachers rated the whole package quite positively (mean=5.51), as they did the "Minder" video (mean=5.72), and the exercises (mean=5.10). The "Thinking Twice" video was also evaluated positively, (mean=4.53), as were the accompanying exercises (mean= 4.71), though these ratings are slightly less favourable than those made for the "Minder" video and notes. There were no differences between teachers as a function of sex, position in school, or subject taught and ratings of the total package or any of the separate parts. Just less than one-half (44.5%) of teachers had devised their own exercises to accompany "Minder", and one third (33.4%) had devised their own exercises to accompany "Thinking Twice".

We ran a series of analyses of variance to identify any variables that might effect teachers' ratings of the package as a whole or the videos and exercises separately. In the first of these, we compared ratings as a function of (a) the way the package was used (with equal emphasis on the two parts, with more emphasis on "Minder", with more emphasis on "Thinking Twice" and with differences between teachers in the school); (b) attendance at drugs education courses and (c) whether or not the school had a coherent drugs policy. Teachers who used both parts of the package equally (mean=6.08) and where there was variability in the school (mean=6.04) rated the package as a whole more favourably then where teachers emphasized "Minder" (mean=5.23) or "Thinking Twice" (mean=5.06); ($F(3, 252) = 8.5, p < .001$). Neither attendance at courses ($F(1, 252) = 0.47$) nor school policy on drugs ($F(1, 252) = 0.01$) affected teachers' ratings. The two-way interaction between use of the package and attendance at courses was, however, significant ($F(7, 252 = 2.09, p < .05$), showing that those who had attended courses and used both parts of the package with equal emphasis rated it most favourably.

A second, related analysis failed to show any significant relationship between ratings of the package and separate components and (a) whether or not other drug education packages were used, and (b) whether or not the school had a policy on drugs.

A third analysis compared ratings of the package as a function of (1) the number of pupils in the school and (2) the type of school (independent, comprehensive, other). Ratings of favourableness to the package were not affected by the number of pupils in the school ($F(2, 373) = 0.13$). However, teachers from comprehensive (state) schools rated the package more favourably (mean=5.78) compared with those from independent (private) schools (mean=5.19), ($F(1, 373) = 5.04, p < .03$).

FIGURE 2.8

Rating of Package (as a whole)

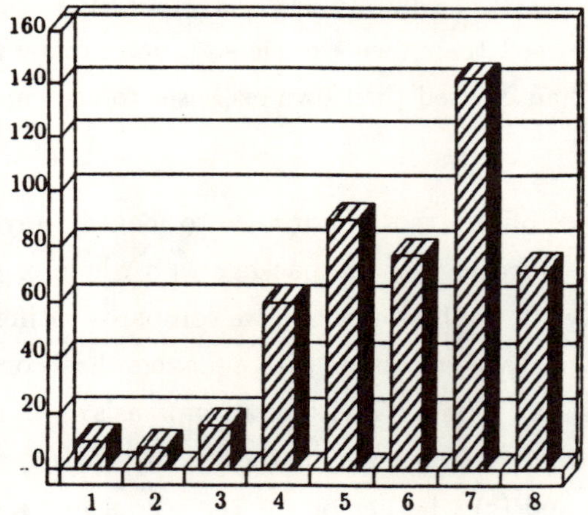

1 - 7 = rating on a 7-point scale ranging from 1 (very unhelpful) to 7 (very helpful)

8 = no answer

FIGURE 2.9

Rating of the two videos

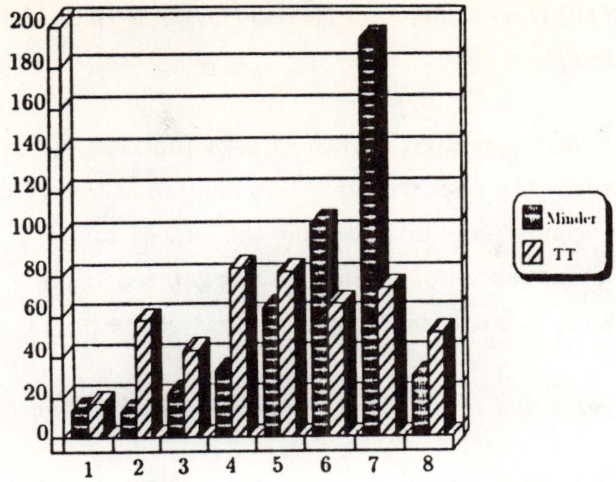

1 - 7 = rating on a 7-point scale ranging from 1 (very unhelpful) to 7 (very helpful)

8 = no answer

FIGURE 2.10

Rating of the exercises / notes

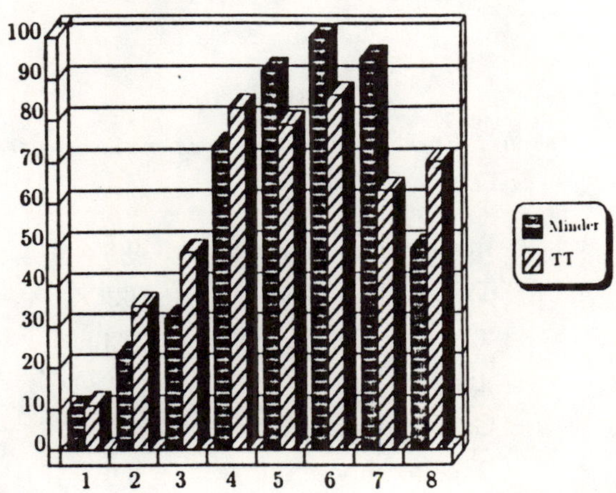

1 - 7 = rating on a 7-point scale ranging from 1 (very unhelpful) to 7 (very helpful)

8 = no answer

A fourth analysis showed that ratings of the whole package were independent of (a) the number of teachers in the school (low; less than 49; high; more than 50) and (2) the teacher- pupil ratio (low; less than 15; medium, 16-18; and high, more than 19)

A fifth analysis compared ratings as a function of (a) the number of teachers who had the package (low, 1-2; medium 3-5 and high, 6 or more); (b) whether or not parents had seen the videos and (c) whether or not sessions for parents about drugs had been organized. None of these variables were significantly related to teachers' ratings of the package.

Teachers' reports and evaluations of other drug education material used

62.0% of teachers used material other than that based on "Double Take" to make up their own drug education courses. The type of material most commonly mentioned is shown in Table 2.1.

School policy on dealing with a pupil found experimenting with drugs

Just under half (41.4 %) of schools had apparently formulated a policy for dealing with pupils found experimenting with drugs. Table 2.2 shows the action that teachers felt they would do if they discovered a pupil experimenting with drugs.

TABLE 2.1

Teachers' reports of other drug material used

	%
Health education leaflets	9.6
TACADE leaflets	16.2
'Chasing the Bandwagon'	3.3
'Its your life'	.7
Government leaflets	1.3
'Free to choose'	3.0
'Just say no'	4.3
Others and more than 1	61.6

TABLE 2.2

Teachers' reports of what they would do if they discovered a pupil experimenting with drugs (percentages)

Inform a parent	73.5	Inform school nurse/dr.	33.9
Inform the family doctor	7.4	Inform LEA	7.4
Inform the police	16.2	Inform EWO	26.1
Contact LEA drug adviser	22.7	Suspend the pupil	6.7
Contact school counsellor	18.1	Discuss with pupils	24.4
Counsel pupil yourself	60.4	Discuss with parents	10.5
Other	27.4	Introduce programme	17.3

A series of Phi-coefficients was then computed to look for relationships between the various actions that teachers might take. The decision to inform a pupil's parents was not significantly related to two items (discussing drugs with all parents and introducing a drug education programme). It related negatively to 'inform school counsellor', but was positively related to all other items. In other words, teachers generally inform a pupil's parents about drug-taking, but if they choose not to, then they are likely to refer the pupil to the school counsellor instead.

Other actions fell into two main clusters. Some teachers opted for a generally hard-line approach, indicated by a tendency to endorse actions involving the police, the local Education Authority and suspending the pupil. Other teachers tended to endorse actions involving the school counsellor, the Local Authority Advisory Teacher for drugs and introducing a drugs education programme for all pupils.

In addition, we conducted a series of χ^2 statistics to look for relationships between each of the individual actions and five other variables. These were (1) school (independent or comprehensive); (2) sex of respondent; (3) position of respondent in school; (4) whether or not the respondent had attended any courses on drugs education and (5) general attitude of respondent.

There were a number of significant associations between the actions which would be taken if a pupil was found experimenting with drugs and the type of school. Respondents from comprehensive schools were more likely to endorse actions involving the Local Authority Advisory Teachers ($\chi^2 = 9.90, p < .01$). Those from independent schools were more likely to endorse actions such as informing the Educational Welfare Officer ($\chi^2 = 26.16, p < .001$), suspending the pupil ($\chi^2 = 28.40, p < .001$) and discussing drugs with all pupils ($\chi^2 = 12.25, p < .001$).

There was only one association between sex of respondent and action that would be taken; male teachers were more likely to inform the police than female teachers ($\chi^2 = 6.15, p < .05$).

We compared teachers in terms of their position in school (head teachers versus other). Head teachers were more likely to inform parents ($\chi^2 = 8.13, p < .01$), inform the school counsellor ($\chi^2 = 9.23, p < .01$) or take some 'other' action ($\chi^2 = 5.32, p < .05$) than other teachers.

Teachers who had attended a drugs course themselves were more likely to contact Local Authority Advisory teachers ($\chi^2 = 11.00, p < .001$) or counsel the pupil themselves ($\chi^2 = 5.15, p < .05$) and less likely to contact Educational Welfare Officers ($\chi^2 = 9.97, p < .01$) or to suspend the pupils ($\chi^2 = 5.49, p < .05$) than teachers who had not attended such courses.

Teachers' personal attitudes to the package had little significant impact on their actions when dealing with a pupil experimenting with drugs. Those with positive attitudes were less likely to inform the Local Education Authority ($\chi^2 = 8.52, p < .05$) and more likely to introduce a drug-education programme ($\chi^2 = 8.51, p < .05$) than teachers with less favourable attitudes to the packages.

Teachers' beliefs about why young people start to take drugs

Teachers rated 20 items concerned with why pupils take drugs each on 7-point scales (from 'definitely no' to 'definitely yes'). These data are shown in Table 2.3.

A principal components analysis on these 20 items yielded six factors. The first, accounting for 18.4% of the variance had the highest loadings on items dealing with *fun/adulthood* (they find it exciting, .74; think it will be fun, .72; want to try something new, .68; want to look grown up, .62 and see adults drinking and smoking, .43). Factor 2 (9.9% of the variance) was

TABLE 2.3

Teachers' beliefs about why pupils take drugs

	Mean	*SD*
Excitement	4.73	1.49
Problems at school	3.21	1.54
Too much publicity	2.91	1.60
Problems at home	4.63	1.50
See adults drinking	4.12	1.97
Fun	5.23	1.43
Parents don't look after them	3.50	1.71
Feel low	4.46	1.46
Bad company	5.79	1.17
Don't think about consequences	5.71	1.28
Pushed into it	5.82	1.00
Want to look grown up	5.01	1.46
Try something new	5.21	1.23
Too much freedom	3.65	1.59
No sense of right and wrong	2.77	1.55
Only the once	5.60	1.35
Bored	5.20	1.41
Feel they won't get a job	3.58	1.63
Get hold of drugs easily	4.86	1.47
Don't know enough about drugs	4.45	1.80

(1 = definitely no; 7 = definitely yes)

an *opportunistic* factor (they tell themselves it will only be once, .61; pushed into it by other young people, .58; feel they won't get a job, .57; they're bored, .53 and they can get hold of drugs too easily, .42). Factor 3 (8.0% of the variance) referred to *problems* (problems at home, .81; feeling low, .71 and problems at school, .69). Factor 4 (7.6% of the variance) centred on *morality* items, (they're given too much freedom, .79; they've no sense of right and wrong, .70; parents don't look after them properly, .55 and there's too much publicity about drugs, .47). Factor 5 (6.5% of the variance) only included one item (they get into *bad company*, .81). Factor 6 (5.2% of the variance) related to *consequences* (they don't know enough about what drugs will do, .80 and they don't think about the consequences, .60).

Teachers' beliefs about how to persuade young people not to take drugs

Teachers rated twelve items concerned with how to persuade young people not to take drugs on a series of 7-point scales (from 'definitely no' to 'definitely yes'). These data are summarized in Table 2.4.

TABLE 2.4

Teachers' beliefs about how to persuade young people not to take drugs

	Mean	*SD*
Make them scared	3.70	2.10
Talk about alcohol	4.81	2.05
Talk about tobacco	4.69	2.03
Talk about coffee	3.56	2.18
Talk about medicine	4.42	2.05
Imagine being offered Heroin	5.62	1.50
Involve parents	5.50	1.35
Practice saying no	6.06	1.30
Talk about problems	6.19	1.13
Help them feel good	6.34	1.02
Help make decisions	6.48	0.88
Imagine what it would be like to be addicted to Heroin	5.78	1.53

(1 = definitely no; 7 = definitely yes)

A principal components analysis on these ratings yielded 3 factors. Factor 1 (34.2% of the variance) related to *talking about other drugs* at the same time (talk about tobacco, .94; talk about alcohol, .93; talk about tea and coffee, .88 and talk about medicines, .83). Factor 2 (20.0% of the variance) seemed to relate most closely to a *decision-making/life-skills* approach (help them feel good about themselves, .87; help them make decisions for themselves, .84; help them talk about personal problems and worries, .79; help them to practice saying no, .66, and involve their parents in drug education, .47). Factor 3 (10.2% of the variance) seemed to combine endorsement of fear-arousal and *role-play* approaches (help them imagine being addicted to heroin, .80; help them imagine being offered heroin, .64; and make them really scared, .53).

Teachers' attitudes and their ratings of 'Double Take'

The principal components analyses reported in the previous sections were used to classify the teachers according to whether they scored high or low on items related to particular factors. Thus, in terms of beliefs about methods of persuasion, teachers were divided into those who agreed to greater or less extents that it was a good idea to *talk about other drugs*, and so on for the other factors. A series of multivariate analyses of variance were then conducted to determine if those scoring high or low on any given factor differed in terms of their evaluations of the package as a whole and/or of its different components. (These evaluations were each on a scale from 1 to 7).

Teachers who agreed more (as opposed to less) with the persuasion strategy of *talking about other drugs* gave more positive evaluations of (i) the package as a whole (means:high, 5.78, low, 5.29; $F(1,323) = 7.56, p < .001$); (ii) the "Minder" video (means: 6.9; 5.48; $F(1,323) = 11.07, p < .001$); (iii) the "Minder" notes (means: 5.44, 4.77; $F(1,323) = 13.19, p < .001$); and (iv) the "Thinking Twice" notes (means: 4.93, 4.54; $F(1,323) = 4.31, p < .04$). However, there were no significant differences in their ratings of the "Thinking Twice" video.

Teachers who showed higher endorsement of a *decision-making/life-skills* strategy gave more favourable evaluations of (i) the package as a whole (means 5.78*vs.* 5.22, $F(1,323) = 9.30, p < .002$), (ii) the "Minder" video (means 6.04 *vs.* 5.45, $F(1,323) = 9.38, p < .002$); (iii) the "Minder" notes (means 5.40 *vs.* 4.73, $F(1,323) = 13.42, p < .001$); (iv) the "Thinking Twice" video (means 4.89 *vs.* 4.36, $F(1,323) = 6.16, p < .02$) and (v) the "Thinking Twice" notes (means 4.90 *vs.* 4.52, $F(1,323), 4.13, p < .04$).

No differences were found in terms of evaluative ratings of the package between teachers who scored higher or lower in terms of their endorsement of *fear-arousal/role-play* strategies. Fewer effects were found in relation to teachers' endorsements of different explanations for adolescent drug-use. The only significant differences observed were associated with the *morality* items. Teachers who agreed more with morality explanations gave *less* favourable ratings of the package as a whole (means 5.31 *vs.* 5.69, $F(1, 323) = 5.68, p < .02$) and of the "Minder" video.

Predicting overall evaluations from specific beliefs

A general evaluative attitude score was calculated for each teacher by simply summating the five separate evaluative ratings considered in the previous section (of the whole package, of each video, and of each set of notes). This general attitude score was then regressed onto the items concerning persuasion strategies and explanations for drug-use. Using a step-wise solution, a multiple R of 0.l41 was obtained after 5 steps. The items identified were:-

(1) imagine being offered heroin (beta = .21, $t = 4.10, p < .001$);

(2) talk about tobacco at the same time as heroin (beta = .19, $t = 3.60, p < .001$);

(3) problems at home (beta = .18, $t = 3.53, p = .001$);

(4) won't get a job (beta = .13, $t = 2.40, p = .02$) and

(5) make decisions for themselves (beta = .11,$t = 2.14, p < .03$).

With a direct solution, there was one other variable that produced a significant beta weight. This was 'excitement' (beta = .14, $t = 2.30, p < .02$).

A separate analysis was then conducted using the same dependent variable (general attitude to the package) but using the mean scores on categories of items ('sub-scales') identified by the previous principal components analyses, rather than the individual items. Using a step-wise solution, a multiple R of .34 was obtained after 3 steps. The predictors included were:-

(1) *'talk about other drugs'* (beta = .23, $t = 4.24, p < .001$);

(2) *'decision-making life-skills'* (beta $= .20, t = 3.70, p < .003$); and

(3) *'problems'* (beta $= -.11, t = 2.17, p < .04$).

With a direct solution, there was one other sub-scale with a significant beta weight: *'morality'*, (beta $= -.11$, $t = -2.10, p < .04$).

Predicting comparative evaluations of "Minder" and "Thinking Twice".

Similar analyses were then conducted using the difference scores computed by subtracting teachers' ratings of "Minder" from their ratings of "Thinking Twice". Using a step-wise solution, a multiple R of .12 was obtained. Only one item entered into the equation — the extent to which teachers felt parents should be involved in drug education (beta = -.12, $t = -2.40, p < .02$), suggesting that teachers who were less keen to involve parents preferred "Minder". A direct solution did not identify any other items with significant beta weights.

Teachers' reasons for not completing the questionnaire

Fortyseven teachers returned their questionnaire or sent letters explaining why they did not feel able or were unwilling to take part in the evaluation.

Discussion

Although we might have hoped for a higher response rate, the overall figure of 56.2% is considerably better than is often reported in postal surveys of this kind. As is always the case in these situations, it is never clear as to why non-respondents chose not to reply. We may speculate that there were a higher proportion of teachers within this group who did not like the approach taken in the package, had decided to use other material rather than "Double Take", or who did not include any systematic drug education in the curriculum at all. However, the fact that there were no differences between our early and late respondents in terms of their ratings of the package or attitudes may perhaps be taken as tentative support for the idea that respondents were not necessarily very different as a group from non-respondents. It may be that teachers did not complete the questionnaire because they felt over-worked or irritated rather than that they felt negative toward the package. In practice, we suspect that many non-respondents had not used the package and felt that they had little comment to make. Certainly some of the very late respondents apologized for the delay and attributed it to the fact that the video was only just being integrated into the curriculum. We also received some letters from teachers explaining that they felt unable to complete the questionnaire because they had not used the package.

Informal chats with teachers suggest that they see alcohol rather than heroin as the drug that produces most problems. Very few teachers reported that individual pupils in the school were known to take drugs, and this can result in a reluctance to introduce the topic into the school. We also found that many schools are still in the process of organizing social and health education courses and the content of the drugs component in particular. They reported large changes in emphasis between the academic years 1985-1986 and 1986-1987, and that they expected to continue to make changes over the following year. In part this must be due to the ever-increasing amount of material available for drugs education. Teachers thinking about organizing such a course are faced with a large selection of programmes, some devised specifically for schools and freely available, some devised for schools but expensive, as well as current affairs programmes that may be highly topical and especially appropriate for older pupils. Since there is as yet no definitive evidence that any one approach is more successful than another, teachers are probably quite justified to base their courses on a selection of available material.

Not only is the content of drugs courses highly variable, so also is the place of this kind of teaching in the curriculum. While independent schools typically approach these issues in biology lessons, or delegate the school matron to hold some informal sessions, the majority of state schools have opted to cover the topic in classes concerned with social education. Yet these differ widely in terms of other topics covered in the same course and the amount of time available. While some schools have a coherent policy on social education over a 3-year period, others have much more restricted programmes.

Two factors suggest that these courses still have rather low status in the curriculum. The first is that the course is rarely examined. Some schools devise informal evaluations on their own course content, but it is rare that pupils work toward a public examination. The second is that few teachers are trained specifically in the kind of teaching that is required of the 'life-skills' approach. It may well be that the kind of style that is required in these courses is distinctly different from the style they adopt when teaching their basic subject. In our study, not quite half the teachers had attended relevant in-service courses. The procedure in most schools seems to be that one teacher becomes responsible for selecting the material to be used, and guides the other teachers in its implementation. The situation is quite different from the way in which more 'respectable' subjects tend to be taught. Often the individual teacher has little idea of what other material may be available, and must rely on advice from colleagues as to how best to organize the class.

There is, in any case, some research evidence to suggest that teachers may be reluctant to take on the teaching of health issues. In the United States, work by Chen & Winder (1983), and Higgins *et al* (1983) has shown that teachers did not see it as their responsibility to teach pupils about the dangers of cigarette smoking. We have found in a related context that teachers are reluctant to discuss issues like illness or death with pupils (Eiser & Town, 1987).

We agree with one teacher, who suggested that teachers needed educating about drugs before pupils. Certainly our results do suggest that teachers' personal attitudes influence their ratings of the package. Those who favour a decision-making approach and do *not* see problems at home as an important factor in why pupils take drugs, favour the 'Minder' over the 'Thinking Twice' video. This suggests that it is necessary to persuade teachers of the value of a decision-making/life-skills approach before the package is likely to meet with their approval and commitment. Those who believe that drug-taking is a response to problems at home or school are less likely to rate the package highly.

It is also worth noting that the package was rarely (if ever) integrated into the curriculum of independent schools. Staff at these schools seem to take the view that (1) drug-taking is not a problem and does not need to be covered and (2) there is so much pressure on curriculum time from examination subjects that 'drugs' cannot be included. Yet it is clear that pupils in these schools are not immune. Again, teachers need to be made aware of their vulnerability before adequate drug-education can take place.

"Double Take" has been quite widely accepted, and it is clear that it can be used very effectively. The combination of video and exercises are an excellent basis for a drugs course with the further advantage that teachers have a choice of approach between "Minder" and "Thinking Twice". In this respect, however, it is unfortunate that the "Thinking Twice" video does not match the "Minder" video in terms of professionalism of technical production. To be maximally effective, however, the programme needs the additional momentum that can only be achieved by promotion and guidance from highly skilled personnel. If videos of this kind are to be used successfully in schools, teachers need back-up and advice from those who are highly experienced in the approach. The success of these videos is dependent on the provision of an adequate number of Advisory Teachers trained in their effective implementation.

3

An observation and evaluation of a course based on "Minder"

Introduction

The aims of this study were (1) to see how the "Double Take" package could be integrated into an existing Social Education Course and (2) to evaluate the effectiveness of the programme in promoting healthy attitudes towards drugs.

The research came about because a local comprehensive invited the Drugs Advisory Teacher to help them set up a drugs programme for 5th year pupils. She alone was responsible for organizing the content of the course, and chose to focus the work on "Minder".

Method

Subjects

The pupils were all enrolled in a comprehensive school about 5 miles outside the city of Exeter. The school caters for a largely rural community, and has approximately 870 pupils, aged between 11 and 18 years. The entire 5th year (15-16 years) was involved in the study. In practice, 112 pupils (66 boys and 46 girls) completed a questionnaire before the start of the course, and 136 pupils (74 boys and 62 girls), including 89 from the previous sample, completed a questionnaire 2 weeks after the end of the course. (Initial testing was carried out during the week before Christmas when many pupils were involved in the end of term activities).

Procedure

Drugs education is taught as part of the Social Education course in the school. This is a 2 year programme. In the fourth year, pupils take courses in 'You and the Law', family and personal relationships, decision-making, careers education and conflict and cooperation. In the fifth year, pupils take courses in job seeking, further education, study skills, drugs, (including alcohol and smoking), contraception, and sexually- transmitted diseases. Each course is the responsibility of one teacher. In the fifth year, pupils are divided into six groups, and rotate between the six courses. The work is not examined. The course on drugs was run separately for two groups of pupils, though the content of the lessons was similar. All these lessons were led by the Local Education Authority Drugs Advisory Teacher, with the regular teacher sitting in and taking a minimal role.

Description of the course

In the first session, it was explained that the aim of the course was not to give facts that were already known about drugs, but to encourage pupils to talk about their feelings and attitudes toward drugs and drug-takers. The class was asked to report the first word they thought of on hearing the word 'drug', and then to write down the names of as many drugs as they could. They then attempted to categorize these as 'legal', 'illegal', 'harmful', or 'useful'. These exercises were used to point out that many drugs had more than one function, and that some substances which were potentially harmful were in fact freely available. Pupils were encouraged to think about how they had reacted when they were first offered a cigarette or alcohol, in order to prepare themselves for how they might react to being offered other drugs. In the second session, pupils viewed the "Minder" video, and worked on two of the exercises published with it. These exercises encouraged pupils to think about their attitudes to some general issues (e.g. whether they felt justified in not paying their fare on a bus if nobody asked for it, or buying cigarettes for someone under age).

In the third session, pupils were shown the first two parts of the video. They were asked their opinions of the main characters, and their understanding of why the characters behaved as they did. The fourth session was devoted to alcohol education and centred on another film called "The Unexpected Guest". In the fifth session, we showed the final part of the "Minder" video. In this part, it becomes clear that two of the boys are taking drugs, and the effect on their character and behaviour was discussed.

Evaluation of the course

Prior to the commencement of the course, all fifth year pupils were administered a brief questionnaire. This covered the following topics:-

(1) *Knowledge of drugs* (in terms of their answers to the question 'What is a drug?' and the number of drugs they could name.)

(2) *Current smoking and drinking habits* (in terms of frequency of smoking and drinking and whom they usually drank with - alone, with parents, or with friends).

(3) *Self-ratings* Pupils rated the statement 'How well do you think you are doing in your school work?' on a 7-point scale from 1 = 'not at all well' to 7 = 'very well indeed'.

(4) *Perceptions of parental behaviour* Pupils rated 8 statements on a series of 7-point scales from 1 = 'never true' to 7 = 'almost always true'. Two such statements were: 'My parents keep changing their minds about what I can and cannot do'. 'My parents' rules don't make much sense'.

(5) *Social competence* Pupils rated ten statements on a series of 7-point scales (from 1 = 'definitely no' to 7 = 'definitely yes'). For example: 'How well do you generally: get on with people your own age; get on with your teachers; get on when you go to new places'.

(6) *Perceived reasons for drug-use* Pupils rated 20 statements (on the same 7-point scales) concerned with why people start to take drugs. For example:

- 'They're having problems at home'.
- 'They tell themselves it will only be the once'.
- 'They find it exciting to take risks'.

The questionnaire used after the course repeated most of the above categories of questions (2,3,4,5, and 6). In addition, we included:-

(7) *Perceptions of the dangerousness of substances* Pupils rated 13 substances (see Table 3) on two 7-point scales. First, each substance was rated as to how addictive it was (where 1 = 'definitely no' and 7 =

'definitely yes' and second each substance was rated as to how likely it was to kill (1 = 'definitely no' and 7 = 'definitely yes').

(8) *Beliefs about how to stop people taking drugs* Pupils rated 10 items concerned with how to stop people taking drugs on 7-point scales as described above. For example:

- 'Make them really scared'.
- 'Talk about alcohol and tobacco at the same time as heroin'.
- 'Help them to make decisions for themselves'.

In addition, pupils in one of the classes that had participated in the drugs programme were asked their opinions of the course. The evaluation consisted of written responses to the following five questions:

(1) What I did not like about these sessions was...;

(2) What I did like was ...;

(3) What I learned is ...;

(4) What I wanted to learn is ...;

(5) These lessons have made me think ...;

The questionnaires are shown in Appendix B.

Results

The analyses will be described under three headings:

(a) those based on data from the first ('before') questionnaire (N=112),

(b) those based on data from the second ('after') questionnaire only (N = 136),

(c) 'before-after' comparisons on those pupils who completed both questionnaires (N=89).

(a) *Analyses of first questionnaire*

Responses to the question 'What is a drug?' were coded in terms of eight categories, as listed in Table 3.1. This table presents the percentages of those responding within each category. (Some subjects' responses were coded in more than one category). Table 3.2 shows the categories of drugs mentioned when pupils were asked to write down as many drugs as they could think of. The mean number of drugs mentioned was 7.18 (the range being 2 to 17. Boys mentioned marginally more drugs than did girls (7.64 *vs.* 6.52, $t = 1.81, p < .1$).

In response to questions about their smoking and drinking behaviour, 60.7% of pupils claimed not to smoke at all. However, 12.5% smoked some days and 25.9% claimed to smoke everyday. Just over one-third (37.5%) claimed never to have been drunk, 20.5% had been drunk once and 40.2% had been really drunk more than once.

Evaluation of the programme

Responses were coded as follows:

(a) *'What I did not like about these sessions was ...'.*

Pupils most commonly complained that 'they knew it all before' (75%). Two pupils did not like all the discussion and the rest had other general complaints (boring).

(b) *'What I did like was ...'.*

Half the pupils specifically stated that they enjoyed the video. 20% enjoyed the discussions, the 'openness' and 'honesty' of the sessions. The rest gave rather general responses (not having to do much work).

(c) *'What I learned is ...'.*

Some pupils (15%) said they had learned never to take drugs. Others mentioned specific facts about drugs that had been learned (20%) and the rest mentioned generally that they had learned 'a lot' about drugs.

TABLE 3.1

Responses to the question "What is a drug?"
Percentages of subjects responding within each category

Category	%
No response	24.1
Alteration of body state	50.0
Alteration of mental state (e.g. makes you feel good)	20.5
Medical (e.g. eases pain)	31.3
Addiction	18.8
Physical harm / death (e.g. kills you)	9.8
Availability / how taken (e.g. get from doctors/sniffed)	0.9
Like smoking / drinking	2.7

TABLE 3.2

Percentages of subjects naming different categories of drugs

Drug	%
No response	17.0
Heroin	86.6
Cocaine	69.6
Solvents	18.8
Amphetamines	43.8
Cannabis	76.8
LSD	70.5
Magic mushrooms	25.9
Hypno-sedatives	7.1
Tranquillizers	4.5
Alcohol	29.5
Tobacco	33.9
Caffeine	27.7

(d) *'What I wanted to learn is ...'*

Half the pupils felt they wanted to know facts about drugs that had not been covered in the course. 20% wanted to learn about sex or AIDS and the rest mentioned irrelevant topics (metalwork, computing).

(e) *'These lessons have made me think ...'*.

Two pupils stated that they had learned it was stupid to smoke, and one claimed to have given up. Half stated that the sessions had made them think more about drugs; 25% felt they would never take drugs.

(b) *Before-after comparisons*

Before considering changes as a result of the intervention, we inspected the data to ascertain the levels of test-retest reliability in subjects' responses, particularly to questions relating to smoking and drinking habits. The 'before' and 'after' measures were strongly related to each other. The item concerning smoking status showed a Kendall's tau of 0.85 between the two measures ($r = 0.92$), the item concerning whether they smoked every day, a tau of 0.74 ($r = 0.81$) and that concerning how often they had been drunk, a tau of 0.76 ($r = 0.81$). Responses to the question concerning whether they ever drunk alone, with others, etc., were similarly stable (*taus* > 0.45 across the five categories). Self-ratings of school performance were also quite stable (tau = 0.57, $r = 0.63$), as were reports of how much pocket money they had to spend (tau= 0.60, $r = 0.74$). Correlations between the two sets of ratings of reasons why young people started to take drugs were significant (rs between 0.25 and 0.55) for all items except one ('because they don't think about the consequences').

A multivariate analysis of variance was then performed on the two sets of 'reasons for starting' ratings. Subjects were classified according to sex, and two other factors: smoking status, with three levels ('never-smokers', 'ex-smokers/triers' and 'current smokers' on the basis of their responses to the second questionnaire), and class-group (the four classes who did not receive the intervention formed one group, the two classes who received the intervention were combined to form the second). There were two 'within subjects' factors: before *vs.* after, and items. This analysis showed that some reasons were more readily endorsed than others overall. (Items: $F(19, 59) = 26.60, p < .001$), and that the ratings tended to be higher on the second questionnaire (Before/after: $F(1, 77) = 16.86, p < .001$.)

The only other significant effect was the Class-group x Before/after x Items interaction, ($F(19, 59) = 2.63, p < .01$). This implies that the intervention may have influenced subjects' views of why young people took drugs, but such effects depended on the specific items. Univariate F-tests showed that the intervention group was more likely ($p < .02$) than the control group to endorse the reason 'Their parents don't look after them properly' before (4.14 *vs.* 3.12) but not after (4.05 *vs.* 3.62) the intervention. Conversely, the intervention group was more likely than the control group to endorse the following statements afterwards but not before: 'They're in the wrong place at the wrong time' (before, 4.14 *vs.* 4.11; after 5.41 *vs.* 4.21, $p < .01$), 'There's too much publicity about drugs' (before 2.65 *vs.* 3.43; after 3.97 *vs.* 2.90, $p < .02$) and 'They're bored' (before 4.56 *vs.* 4.46; after 5.84 *vs.* 4.37, $p < .001$) afterwards but not before (4.14 *vs.* 4.11; 2.65 *vs.* 3.43, and 4.56 *vs.* 4.46 respectively).

(c) *Analyses of second questionnaire: ratings of dangerousness.*

In view of the larger number of subjects completing the second questionnaire, the larger number of items included, and the lack of any class-group differences on relevant 'before' measures, the remaining analyses were conducted on the 'after' measures only.

We first considered the ratings of how addictive and likely to kill were the 13 different substances. A multivariate analysis of variance was performed with sex, smoking status and class-group as 'between subjects' factors, and two 'within subjects' factors: ratings of addictiveness *vs.* likelihood to kill, and substances. This yielded a significant main effect for Class-group, $F(1, 118) = 5.06, p < .05$, indicating that the intervention group evaluated the substances more negatively overall. This effect was more marked for females (Sex x Class-group, $F(1, 118) = 5.84, p < .02$).

The Addictive/kill main effect was highly significant, $F(1, 118) = 49.47$, $p < .001$, indicating that the substances were seen overall as more addictive than likely to kill. The Substance main effect was highly significant, $F(12, 107) = 125.71, p < .001$, reflecting differences in the perceived dangerousness of the different substances. The Sex x Substance interaction was significant, $F(12, 107) = 2.23, p < .02$, (females rated cannabis more negatively, and chocolate as more addictive), as was the Class-group x Substance interaction $F(12, 107) = 27.94, p < .001$. The Addictive/kill substance interaction ($F(12,107) = 27.94, p < .001$) and the Class-group x Addictive/kill x Substance interaction, $F(12,107) = 2.50, p < .01$, were the only other effects to achieve significance. The means for each item on each scale for the intervention and control groups are shown in Table 3.3. Univariate F-tests showed that beer was rated as significantly more addictive ($F(1,118) = 3.96, p < .05$) and likely to kill ($F(1,118) = 8.99, p < .01$) by the intervention than by the control group.

TABLE 3.3

Mean ratings by control and intervention groups of how addictive and likely to kill were different substances (7-point scales)

	Addictive		*'Likely*	*to kill'*
Class-group:	Control	Intervention	Control	Intervention
Substance				
Chocolate	3.05	3.43	1.54	1.53
Tranquillizers	5.99	6.44	5.72	5.56
Tea/coffee	4.72	5.28	2.16	1.71
Cigarettes	6.62	6.84	6.39	6.63
Heroin	6.80	6.98	6.99	6.97
Beer	5.52	6.01	4.83	5.80
Spirits	6.03	6.41	5.79	6.28
Glue/Solvents	6.44	6.70	6.69	6.56
Cocaine	6.80	6.82	6.88	6.83
Sleeping Pills	5.62	5.92	6.17	6.36
Vitamin Pills	3.77	4.46	3.27	4.05
LSD	6.48	6.58	6.58	6.83
Cannabis	6.14	6.35	6.08	6.25
N	87	43	87	43

A series of principal components analyses were then performed, (with varimax rotation) the first being on the ratings of addictiveness. This yielded a strong first factor, accounting for 43.8% of the variance, with highest loadings on solvents, .81; cigarettes, .77; spirits, .75; beer, .71; cocaine, .67; heroin, .66; sleeping pills, .62; and tranquillizers, .60. A second factor (14.2% of the variance) related mainly to illegal drugs (cannabis, .84; LSD, .66; heroin, .59; and cocaine, .58). A third factor (8.2% of the variance) comprised chocolate, .78; tea/coffee, .71 and vitamin pills, .63.

An equivalent analysis on the 'kill' ratings yielded a somewhat different structure with four factors , Factor 1 (27.5% of the variance) included spirits, .85; solvents, .67; beer, .66; cigarettes, .66, sleeping pills, .62; and LSD, .51, (heroin had a zero loading). Factor 2 (12.2% of the variance) included cannabis, .75; vitamin pills, .75 and tranquillizers, .52. Factor 3(11.2% of the variance) comprised tea/coffee, .83; and chocolate, .83. Finally, Factor 4 related almost exclusively to heroin, .86; and cocaine, .68.

(d) *Beliefs about persuasion*

A principal components analysis on subjects' ratings of how best 'to persuade young people not to try drugs like heroin' yielded three factors. Factor 1 (34.3% of the variance) seemed to relate most closely to endorsement of a decision-making/ life-skills approach (Help them to feel good about themselves, .85; Help them to talk about their personal problems and worries, .82; Help them to make decisions for themselves, .80; and Give them as much information as possible, .64). Factor 2 (17.2% of the variance) related to talking about other kinds of drugs 'at the same time as heroin', specifically tea/coffee, .82; medicine, .81; and alcohol and tobacco, .68. Factor 3 (11.2% of the variance) seemed to combine endorsement of fear-arousal and 'role-play' approaches ('Make them really scared', .71; 'Help them to practise saying no', .71; and 'Help them to imagine being offered heroin', .55).

(e) *Reasons why young people start taking drugs*

A principal components analysis on these 20 items yielded five factors. The first, accounting for 28.8% of the variance, had the highest loadings on items dealing with experimentation ('They want to try something new', .71; 'They think it will be fun',.68; 'They find it exciting to take risks;, .68; 'They tell themselves it will only be once', .64; 'They're pushed into it by other young people', .64; 'They don't think about the consequences', .64.) Factor 2 (9.8% of the variance) related to themes of morality/disipline (e.g. 'They're given too much freedom', .73; 'They've no sense of right or wrong', .72; 'Their parents don't look after them properly', .54). Factor 3 (8.3% of the variance) referred to problems ('They're having problems at home', .74; 'They're feeling low at the time', .68; and 'They're having problems at school', .67). Factor 4 (6.1% of the variance) centred on anticipation of adulthood ('They want to look grown up', .81; 'They see adults drinking and smoking', .77; 'They feel they won't get a job', .45). Finally, Factor 5 (5.5% of the variance) related most strongly to two items: 'There's too much publicity about drugs', .82, and 'They're bored', .62.

(f) *Social competence*

Three factors were derived from a principal components analysis of the ten self-ratings of 'social competence'. Factor 1 (31.8% of the variance) related to new situations, and peers ('Get on when you meet people you don't know', .88; 'Get on when you go to new places', .86; and 'Get on with people of your own age', .68). Factor 2 (15.8% of the variance) related to interactions with adults ('Get on with your teachers', .83, 'Get on with your parents', .81; 'Get on with adults', .58; this last item also loading .42 on Factor 1). Factor 3 (12.2% of the variance) comprised the remaining four items dealing with general autonomous maturity, ('Make decisions for yourself'. .72; 'Say "no" when you feel you shouldn't do something', .68; 'Cheer yourself up when you feel low', .62; and 'Understand other people's feelings', .57). A reliability analysis of the extent to which all ten items could be summated to give a single scale yielded a Cronbach's alpha of .74.

(g) *Relationships with parents*

The eight item scale concerning relationships with parents had adequate internal consistency as an additive scale (Cronbach's alpha = .75) with item 2 being scored in the reverse direction. A principal components analysis on these items, however, distinguished two factors, accounting respectively for 38.8% and 13.6% of the variance. Factor 1 included five of the eight items dealing most closely with parental discipline (e.g. 'My parents don't allow me enough freedom to do what I want to do', .78), whereas Factor 2 comprised the remaining three items dealing more with parental attention/control ('I decide things for myself even when my parents disagree with me', .82; 'My parents aren't interested in my problems and the decisions I have to make', .59; and (with reversed scoring) 'My parents always know where I am and what I'm doing', .38).

(h) *Analyses of subscale scores*

In order to consider the results of the above analyses in relation to each other, we first calculated a number of 'subscale' scores (essentially, unweighted factor scores) based on the items loading most highly on the factors revealed by the last four principal components analyses described. Thus, three subscales were derived from the ratings of best methods of persuasion, with the first subscale (Persuasion 1: decisions/life-skills) being the mean of the four items loading most strongly on Factor 1, the second subscale being the mean of the three items loading most strongly on Factor 2, and so on for all four analyses, to give a total of 13 subscale scores for each subject.

A stepwise discriminant analysis was then performed (using the method of maximizing the change in Rao's V) to attempt to differentiate the control and intervention groups on the basis of these scores. A further item - subjects' self-ratings of how well they were doing in their school work - was added to the list of discriminating variables. This analysis is summarized in Table 3.4. Although nine variables entered the analysis, the most important discriminating variable is the Reasons 5 sub-scale. In other words, subjects in the intervention group were more likely to identify publicity and boredom as reasons why young people started taking drugs. In terms of univariate differences between the means, the intervention group was also more likely to attribute drug-taking to 'problems' (Reasons 3). In terms of trends suggested by the correlations between each discriminating variable and the discriminant function, compared with the controls the intervention subjects were somewhat more in favour of talking about other drugs at the same time as heroin (Persuasion 2) - which was indeed a theme of the intervention programme - but rated their own social competence lower on items relating to autonomy/maturity. This (together with the weak *negative* correlation with Persuasion 1: decisions/life-skills) goes rather against what one might have expected from an intervention based partly on a 'life-skills' approach.

TABLE 3.4

Discriminant analysis to predict class-group membership from sub-scale scores

Discriminating Variable	Means: Control (N=84)	Means: Intervention (N=41)	Correlation with Canonical Discriminant Function	Univariate F (1,123)	Step entered	Change in Rao's V
Reason 5: publicity/bored	3.58	4.63	0.71	17.91***	1	17.91***
Competence 3: autonomy/maturity	5.58	5.32	-0.27	2.59	2	2.73
Persuasion 2: talk about other drugs	3.78	4.16	0.28	2.79	3	1.86
School work	4.92	5.07	0.14	<1	4	2.15
Persuasion 1: decisions/life-skills	5.85	5.73	-0.10	1.20	5	1.74
Persuasion 3: scare/role-play	5.03	5.24	0.15	<1	6	3.61
Reasons 2: morality/discipline	4.62	4.69	0.05	<1	7	2.47
Reasons 3: problems	4.79	5.25	0.36	4.56*	8	1.65
Competence 2: adults	5.62	5.72	0.09	<1	9	1.47
Reasons 1: experimentation	5.59	5.78	0.16	<1	–	–
Reasons 4: anticipation of adulthood	4.44	4.78	0.11	1.76		
Competence 1: new situations	5.46	5.48	-0.11	<1		
Parents 2: lack of attention	2.29	2.33	-0.11	<1		
Parents 1: lack of rules/consistency	2.36	2.44	.00	<1		
Canonical discriminant function at group means	-0.37	0.76				

* $p < .05$ *** $p < .001$

TABLE 3.5

Multiple regression analyses to predict each persuasion subscale score from the five Reasons subscales.

Dependent variable:	Persuasion 1 (Decisions/life-skills) Beta	t	Persuasion 2 (Talk about other drugs) Beta	t	Persuasion 3 (Scare/role play) Beta	t
Reasons 1: experimentation	0.34	3.63***	0.27	2.74**	0.21	2.07*
Reasons 2: morality/discipline	−0.08	−0.75	−0.19	−1.78	0.22	1.99*
Reasons 3: problems	0.35	3.57***	0.19	1.79	0.03	0.28
Reasons 4: anticipation of adulthood	0.05	0.58	0.23	2.26*	0.09	0.89
Reasons 5: publicity/bored	−0.12	−1.42	−0.04	−0.39	−0.15	−1.66
Adjusted R^2	0.24		0.14		0.13	
$F(5,119)$	8.71***		5.10***		4.78***	

* $p < .05$, ** $p < .01$, *** $p < .001$

An equivalent analysis to discriminate males from females on the basis of the same variables showed few differences, with only four items entering the analysis, and only one of these yielding a significant univariate difference on the group means. This was Persuasion 1: decisions/life-skills, and showed that males were less enthusiastic about this approach to persuasion than were females (subscale means were 5.59 and 6.08; $F(1,123) = 7.32, p < .01$). The other variables entering the analysis were Persuasion 3: scare/role-play; Parents 2: lack of attention; and School work. Males showed slightly higher mean scores on all these variables.

Two further analyses were conducted using the same discriminating variables to predict smoking and drinking status. Smoking status, in terms of the three groups Never-smokers (N=32), Ex-smokers/triers (N=57) and Smokers (N=36), related significantly to three variables in terms of univariate mean differences. These were School work (means: 5.41, 5.12 and 4.33;

$F(2,122) = 14.94, p < .001$) Competence 2:adults (means:6.11, 5.74 and 5.10; $F(2,122) = 8.94, p < .01$) and Parents 2: lack of attention (means:2.04, 2.29, 2.56; $F = 4.93, p < .01$), the last of these not being among the first six variables entered in the stepwise analysis. Thus smokers felt they were doing worse at school, got on worse with parents, teachers and adults, and saw their parents as giving them greater license. The analysis was limited to a single discriminant function, which yielded values of 0.58, 0.25 and -0.91 at the group means. In other words, the differences between the two groups of 'non-smokers' (never-smokers and those who had tried smoking once or twice and/or given it up) were less, overall, than those between either of these two groups and those who were currently smoking.

Drinking status was defined in terms of those who responded 'never' (N=45) 'only once' (N=27) and 'more than once' (N=53) to the question 'Have you ever got really drunk?' The differences were smaller than those related to smoking status, but with the same three variables being the only ones to show significant univariate mean differences, i.e. School work (means: 5.22, 5.19, 4.64; $F(2,122) = 5.88, p < .01$), Parents 2: lack of attention (means: 2.08, 2.26, 2.52, $F(2,122) = 5.13, p < .01$) and Competence 2: adults (means: 5.92, 5.80, 5.35; $F(2,122) = 3.90, p < .05$). As in the previous analysis, the 'never' and 'only once' groups were more similar to each other than to those who had got drunk 'more than once', in terms of the first discriminant function (means: -0.42, -0.26, 0.49). As may be expected, drinking and smoking status were highly associated. The number of 'never' 'only once' and 'more than once' drinkers were 20, 8 and 7 among the never-smokers; 25, 15 and 20 among the ex-smokers/triers, and 4, 7 and 30 among the smokers; χ^2 (4) = 28.04, $p < .001$, Kendall's tau = 0.39, $p < .001$. The association between drinking status and sex was also significant with the frequencies within the respective drinking groups being 19, 15 and 40 for boys and 30, 15 and 17 for girls; χ^2 (2) = 10.78, $p < .001$, Kendall's tau= -0.30, $p < .001$. The association between smoking status and sex, however, was non-significant (χ^2 (2) = 0.65).

Finally, we considered how subjects' views on best methods of persuasion could be predicted from their ratings of the reasons why young people might start taking drugs. Multiple regression analyses were conducted, with each of the three Persuasion subscale scores in turn as dependent variables, and the five Reasons subscale scores as predictors. These are summarized in Table 3.5. As may be seen, Reasons 1: experimentation was a significant predictor of all three Persuasion subscales. In addition, though, attribution of drug-taking to 'problems' (Reasons 3) predicted a favourable attitude towards decision-making and life-skills themes (Persuasion 1); attribution to 'anticipation of adulthood' (Reasons 4) predicted a favourable attitude towards talking about other drugs (Persuasion 2) - such as those taken by adults; and attribution to 'lax morality' or 'discipline' (Reasons 2) predicted a more favourable attitude towards scare/role play approaches (Persuasion 3).

Discussion

The purpose of this study was essentially exploratory, looking at how a 'life-skills' programme was integrated with the curriculum, and received by teachers and pupils, rather than being a formal evaluation. Nevertheless, we were able to identify some very positive effects of the programme on pupils' attitudes.

We would like to consider first, however, some of the difficulties that were encountered in conducting this study. Some were practical and may have been specific to this study. For example, the timing of when the evaluations were made was problematic. The pre-teaching questionnaire had to be administered the week before Christmas, which significantly reduced the number of complete responses. The post-teaching questionnaire was not administered until 2 weeks after the course (with a holiday in between) by which time pupils had been moved to different teaching groups.

Other problems related to the structure of the Social Education course at the school, of which drugs education was a one-sixth component. Since the school had not yet developed a coherent drugs policy, any number of teachers had discussed drugs with the pupils in the past, and it was almost impossible to tell how well-informed they were before our sessions. The result was that some of the pupils felt they knew the 'facts' about drugs. Although it was stressed at the beginning of the course that the purpose was to make them think, let them talk and develop their own attitudes, pupils clearly found the novel approach difficult. Many pupils themselves believe that school is where you learn 'hard facts' and they are inclined to regard any alternative approach as a soft option. In implementing this kind of approach in a school, educators need to take account of the wide disparities between their goals and pupils' other experiences.

A related problem is that of teacher attitudes. As discussed in the previous chapter some teachers may still be reluctant to take on 'health' teaching (Chen & Winder, 1983; Higgins, Dunn & Warmack, 1983). This reluctance may well be even greater where teachers are expected to adopt a teaching style which is markedly different from their more 'tried and tested' techniques. Indeed, it is one problem of the life-skills approach that it is relatively expensive, both in terms of training teachers and in terms of curriculum time (Connell, Turner & Mason, 1985). In the study by Connell *et al.* (1985), for example, it was found that 40 or 50 hours of classroom time were required to produce stable effects on knowledge, attitudes and smoking practices.

In evaluating the effects of this programme, it needs to be noted that our 'teacher' was highly trained in its implementation, motivated and enthusiastic. As has been noted before, it can be difficult to interpret the real value of a programme which may be dependent as much on the skill of the teacher as the content of the programme (Cleary *et al.*, 1986). We are aware of this problem, and in the following study we try to assess how the programme can be integrated in schools which do not have access to such skilled personnel.

Given the practical difficulties encountered in this study, it is perhaps heartening to find some attitude changes in the desired direction following the teaching programme, although these are of course over a very short time period. In particular, pupils who had experienced the life-skills programme evaluated some substances more negatively than those who had not experienced the teaching. The finding that this effect was especially pronounced for girls bears replication. However it may well be that girls are more receptive to this type of approach given their socialization experiences. Indeed there is some evidence for this in the discriminant analysis reported. More surprising was the finding that smokers and non-smokers did not differ in their beliefs about why people start to take heroin or in their ratings of addictiveness of different substances.

There are two areas in which the programme appears to be less successful. The first is in encouraging pupils to think about heroin and other hard drugs in relation to the more acceptable and/or legal ones. Factor analyses showed that even after the life-skills programme, pupils distinguished heroin from the legal drugs both in terms of addictiveness and degree to which it could kill. Many teachers, too, express reservations about convincing pupils to think about their experience with legal drugs when discussing illegal ones. This message may yet prove to be the most difficult one for teachers and pupils to accept.

The second area of concern relates to the findings of the discriminant analysis, comparing subscale scores of pupils in the intervention and control groups. Those in the intervention group were more likely to identify publicity and boredom as reasons why young people start to take drugs. They were also more likely to attribute drug-taking to 'problems', and were somewhat more in favour of talking about other drugs at the same time as heroin - both themes of the intervention programme. What is difficult to reconcile with the 'life-skills' approach is the finding that the intervention group rated their own social competence lower on items relating to autonomy and maturity. We would like to speculate that the intervention group had become more *aware* of these issues as a result of exposure to new ideas in the course, rather than genuinely becoming less autonomous.

What is clear is that the degree to which subjects favour different approaches to drug-education is dependent on their beliefs about the causes of drug-taking. We identified three approaches to persuading people to stop taking heroin; life-skills/decision-making, 'talk about other drugs', and fear/ role-playing. While a belief that people take drugs in order to 'experiment' was related to all three factors, there were other more interesting differences. Subjects who favoured a 'life-skills' approach to education also tended to believe that people took drugs because they were experiencing 'problems'. Those who favoured an approach in which illicit drugs were talked about in context with other legal drugs tended to believe that young people took drugs as a reflection and anticipation of adult behaviour. Finally, those who favoured a fear/role-play approach to education believed that those who take drugs lack morality and discipline.

These findings are suggestive of a link between an individual's beliefs about why people take drugs on the one hand and about the type of education that is likely to be most successful on the other. The argument that we should match health education (in the widest sense) to an individual's beliefs is not new (cf Michela & Contento, 1984). Future research needs to address the question of whether or not matching drug education programmes to an individual's belief system is more successful than offering a single approach to all students.

4

A second evaluation of "Double Take" in a local school

Introduction

The aims of this third study are similar to those described in the introduction to the previous chapter. An opportunity arose to evaluate a drugs prevention programme in a local school. Although pupils were shown the "Minder" video, most of the course was centred on "Thinking Twice". We wanted to see if some of the desired changes in attitudes reported in the last study could be replicated. Although the evaluations not directly comparable, we were interested in whether the impact of a "Thinking Twice" based programme differed from one based on "Minder".

A second purpose was to see how well the programme could be implemented in a school setting where some of the teachers were not highly skilled in the use of the package, and no outside expertise was called in.

Method

The School

The school is a comprehensive, serving an essentially rural population. There are 798 pupils, aged between 11 and 18 years. It is similar to the previous school in terms of its location, age range and social class distribution of pupils.

The pupils

The entire 4th year was involved in the drugs programme (age range 14 to 15 years). 124 pupils completed the questionnaire prior to the course;

147 pupils completed the questionnaire after the course, and 108 pupils completed both questionnaires.

Organization of the social education course

Pupils were divided into 8 groups with about 20 pupils in each group. The drugs programme lasted for 4 weeks (i.e. 4 double periods). One teacher was primarily responsible for the organization of the content of the course, but within this framework each of the 8 teachers made slight changes in emphasis as they wished. All pupils therefore experienced 4 weeks (4 sessions of 1 hour 10 minutes duration) of drug education based on "Minder" and/or "Thinking Twice".

Description of the drugs course

All pupils saw both videos. The "Minder" film tended to be shown once only, with follow-up work organized around one of the worksheets concerned with value judgements. "Thinking Twice" was shown straight through and in separate parts on other occasions. No other videos were shown to pupils.

Procedure

Pupils are divided into tutorial groups (essentially small classes) and for practical reasons the questionnaires were distributed in those sessions. Pupils are divided into different groups for Social Education classes. The questionnaire was introduced as a survey into attitudes towards drugs held by young people. Tutors were asked to impress on pupils that their answers were confidential; that they were to work alone and not leave out any questions. They were also asked to explain to pupils how to use the 7-point rating scales.

The drugs course then took place in 4 sessions over a 2 week period. A few days after the end of the course, follow-up questionnaires were again distributed to pupils by the tutors. In addition, we collected some information from the teachers of the Social Education course as to the exact content of their courses.

Questionnaire

The questionnaire included the following items:-

(1) Perceptions of the dangerousness of substances.

(2) Perceived reasons for drug-use.

(3) Beliefs about how to stop people taking drugs.

(4) Beliefs about who is the most suitable person to teach people about drugs.

Results

(a) *Before-after comparisons*

Before considering changes as a result of the intervention, we inspected the data to ascertain the levels of test-retest reliability in subjects' responses. The 'before' and 'after' measures were strongly related to each other. Correlations between the two sets of ratings of addictiveness of substances were significant (*r*s between .26 and .54) apart from heroin ($r = .10$). Correlations between the two sets of ratings of 'likely to kill' on the 13 substances were all significant (*r*s between .21 and .54). Correlations between ratings of 'why people start to take drugs' were significant, apart from ratings of 'they're pushed into it by other young people' and 'they're having problems at home'. Finally, all correlations between ratings of 'how to persuade others not to take drugs' were significant (*r*s between .20 and .47).

(b) *Perceptions of the dangerousness of substances*

We first considered the ratings of how addictive and likely to kill were the 13 substances. A multivariate analysis of variance was performed with sex and age as 'between subjects' factors, and three 'within subjects' factors; before-after, ratings of addictiveness *vs.* likelihood to kill and substances. There was no overall before-after main effect ($F = .24, ns$). The main effect for substance was significant ($F(12,68) = 85.03$, $p < .001$) as was the addictive/kill main effect, ($F(1,79) = 40.78$, $p < .001$). Substances were therefore seen to be more addictive than killing, though this difference was in itself dependent on particular substances (addictive/kill x substance interaction, ($F(12,68) = 17.09, p < .001$).

In addition, there was a significant before-after x substance interaction ($F(12,68) = 6.89, p < .001$) showing that changes in perceived dangerousness of substances after the course were more attributable to some substances than others. A series of independent t-tests showed that the most significant changes related to perceived increased addictiveness of tea or coffee and beer, and decreased addictiveness of glue, cocaine and cannabis. With regard to 'kill' ratings, chocolate and tea/coffee and vitamin pills were all seen to be more killing after the course and heroin, cocaine, cannabis and cigarettes as less killing. These data are summarized in Table 4.1.

TABLE 4.1

Changes in the addictiveness and likely to kill ratings before and after the 'life-skills' course

	Addictiveness			*'Likely to kill'*		
Substance	*before*	*after*	t	*before*	*after*	t
chocolate	3.07	3.51	1.90	1.76	2.06	1.97
tranquillizers	5.76	5.85	0.53	5.17	5.20	0.18
tea/coffee	4.24	5.23	4.64***	1.87	2.99	6.20***
cigarettes	6.69	6.62	−0.81	6.58	6.30	−2.60*
heroin	6.87	6.69	−1.76	6.89	6.58	−3.21*
beer	5.38	5.76	2.34*	4.74	5.04	1.79
spirits	6.09	6.21	0.96	5.86	6.01	1.10
glue	6.47	5.90	−3.61***	6.47	6.28	−1.71
cocaine	6.67	6.23	−3.70***	6.65	6.20	−3.82***
sleeping pills	5.41	1.68	1.68	5.67	5.53	−0.90
vitamin pills	3.44	3.82	1.77	2.73	3.33	3.66***
LSD	5.99	5.67	−1.83	6.07	5.76	−1.83
cannabis	6.42	5.93	−3.08*	6.25	5.81	−2.95*

$***p < .001$ $\quad *p < .05$

(c) *Perceived reasons for drug-use*

A multivariate analysis of variance was performed on the two sets of 'reasons for starting to take drugs' ratings. Subjects were classified according to sex and age (14 or 15 years). There were two 'within subjects' factors: before-after, and items. This analysis showed that some items were more readily endorsed overall (Items: $F(19,75) = 32.3, p < .001$). In addition, there was a significant before-after x items interaction, ($F(19,75) = 2.37, p < .04$). A series of t -tests showed that, after the course, pupils were more likely to endorse the following statements:

'They want to try something new' ($t = -2.47, p < .02$, means = 5.31 and 5.64);

'They're in the wrong place at the wrong time' ($t = -.32$, $p < .001$, means = 4.31 and 4.99); and

'There's too much publicity about drugs' ($t = -.2.33, p < .02$, means = 2.80 and 3.28).

(d) *Beliefs about how to stop people taking drugs*

A second multivariate analysis of variance was then conducted on the two sets of 'how to persuade people not to take drugs' ratings. Again subjects were classified according to sex and age. Again, some items were more readily endorsed than others ($F(9,83) = 62.9$, $p < .001$) but this was also dependent on the sex of respondents, (sex x items interaction, ($F(9,83) = 2.33$, $p < .02$). There was also a significant before-after x items interaction ($F(9,83) = 7.86, p < .001$). A series of t-tests showed that, after the course, pupils were more likely to endorse the following items:-

'Talk about tea and coffee at the same time as heroin' ($t = -5.75$, $p < .001$, means = 2.25 and 3.45); and

'Help them to imagine being offered heroin' ($t = -3.66$, $p < .001$, means = 5.02 and 5.73).

They were also less likely to endorse these items:-

'Make them really scared' $t = 3.66$, $p < .001$, means = 5.06 and 4.34),

'Help them talk about personal problems and worries' $t = 2.15, p < .03$, means = 5.55 and 5.18),

'Help them to feel good about themselves' ($t = 2.14$, $p < .04$, means = 5.57 and 5.22), and

'Help them to make decisions for themselves' ($t = 2.02$, $p < .05$, means = 5.87 and 5.57).

(e) *Beliefs about who is the most suitable person to teach young people about drugs*

A third multivariate analysis of variance was conducted on the two sets of ratings concerned with 'the best person to teach young people about drugs'. This yielded a significant main effect for items ($F(5,95) = 52.75$, $p < .001$) suggesting that some people were seen as more appropriate overall. There were some differences between boys and girls in whom they perceived to be the most suitable people to give drugs education ($F(5,95) = 2.84$, $p < .02$). Again there was a significant before-after x items interaction ($F(1,98) = 12.11$,)$p < .001$). Pupils were, if anything, more likely after the course to endorse that such teaching should be carried out by ex-drug addicts (means = 6.39 and 6.44, ns) teachers ($t = -3.23$, $p < .002$, means = 3.91 and 4.50) and the police ($t = -.455$, $p < .001$, means = 4.01 and 4.88), but less likely to agree that parents ($t = 3.31$, $p < .001$, means = 4.11 and 3.55), doctors (means = 6.04 and 5.71, ns) and nurses (means = 5.25 and 4.98, ns) should do this kind of teaching.

Discussion

The purpose of this study was two-fold. In part, we were interested in the impact of a programme focused on "Thinking Twice" and whether this could be used to change pupils' attitudes to drugs. In part, too, we were interested in how the programme could be implemented by a group of teachers who did not have the extensive training with the material as the Drugs Advisory Teacher who was involved in the previous study.

Despite the fact that the teachers in this study had not all had any special training in administering the programme, we did find some effects in the desired direction. One of the themes of "Thinking Twice" is to encourage pupils to think about legal and illegal drugs on a continuum. Certainly there was evidence that pupils recognized that substances like coffee and beer were addictive as a result of the programme. Unfortunately, some other substances were seen to be less addictive afterwards - glue, cocaine and cannabis. Heroin, cocaine and cannabis were perceived as less likely to kill after the teaching. The programme appears to succeed in persuading pupils of the potential danger of common substances, but at the expense of making some more dangerous substances seem to be less so.

There was also evidence of some attitude changes. After the course, pupils were more likely to agree that people started to take drugs 'to try something new', 'because they're in the wrong place at the wrong time', and 'because there's too much publicity about drugs'. With respect to their beliefs about how to stop people taking drugs, pupils rated 'talk about tea and coffee at the same time as heroin' and 'help them to imagine being offered heroin' more highly. These were very much central issues of the course. At the same time, pupils rated less favourably 'make them really scared'. What is more difficult to explain is that pupils also rated items concerned with decision-making and life-skills generally more negatively. Judging from their ratings, pupils like learning about illicit drugs in relation to legal ones, but they appear less happy with the 'life-skills' element of the course. This may reflect the fact that pupils are not generally expected to express their opinions or discuss complex issues in schools. The success of the 'life-skills' approach may unfortunately be limited by its novelty. Pupils may need to learn how to operate in small discussion groups. Opportunities for this kind of learning in school are almost negligible and consequently pupils are likely to remain as suspicious of the approach as many of their teachers.

The results of the previous study together with these data suggest that programmes based on "Minder" or "Thinking Twice" each have merits. The impact of the "Thinking Twice" programme appears less dramatic. However, this was not a controlled evaluation, and a number of factors differentiated the two situations. First, in the previous study, the drugs course was organized by the Drugs Advisory Teacher who was highly skilled in the use of the material. In contrast, in this present study, the programme was implemented by eight individual teachers, none of whom had any previous experience w'th the programme. Second, the "Thinking Twice" programme was shorter, based on four teaching sessions compared with five in the previous school. Third, the pupils in this study were one year younger. Although these data do not provide any systematic evidence about the appeal of the programme to different age-groups, it may be that older pupils can benefit significantly more from decision-making approaches to education than younger ones.

5

An experimental investigation of pupils' responses to "Minder" and "Thinking Twice"

Introduction

The results of the previous two studies provide some evidence that the impact of the two films on pupils' attitudes to drugs may not be identical. However, neither of these studies was set up to examine this question directly. In this fourth study, we attempted to compare the immediate impact of the two films on pupils' perceptions of the addictiveness and dangerousness of drugs, on their beliefs about why people take drugs and on their drug-related knowledge.

Video-films are increasingly being used to teach children about a variety of issues. In particular, there have been a number of videos produced to prepare children for minor surgery and hospitalization (Melamed & Siegel, 1975), induction of anesthesia (Vernon & Bailey, 1974) and dental treatment (Adelson & Goldfried, 1970; Machen & Johnson, 1974). Others have used videos to teach children how to cope with sexual abuse (Saslawsky & Wertele, 1986) or to change attitudes towards handicapped peers (Westervelt, Brantley & Ware, 1983; Armstrong, Rosenbaum & King, 1987).

Despite the numbers of films produced, there have been surprisingly few evaluations. Those that have been reported tend to evaluate the success of the film against some other teaching method, typically the traditional lecture. Peterson and Ridley-Johnson, (1984), for example, compared the academic lecture with a film about hospitalization in terms of the effects on children's attitudes and hospital-related knowledge. While both methods succeeded in reducing children's fears about what goes on in hospitals, only the traditional lecture resulted in a measurable increase in knowledge. Westervelt, Brantley and Ware (1983) evaluated a film which emphasized similarities between handicapped and able-bodied school-children. They reported that the film had some positive effects in improving children's attitudes to the handicapped. However, the effects were similar whether children were simply shown the film or whether they participated in a teacher-led discussion in addition to viewing the film.

There has been very little acknowledgement in the literature of whether the impact of the film is at all variable depending on its particular content. The development of most videos is based on some application of Social Learning Theory (Bandura, 1977) and the assumption is that by observing others behave in a particular way, children will adopt similar desired behaviour. Thus, in the films developed for children going to hospital, it is hypothesized that those who view a child coping successfully with the experience (i.e. not crying) will cope successfully themselves. There has been a distinction made between 'coping' and 'mastery' models, and some evidence that the 'mastery' model (in which a child is initially stressed but overcomes this fear in the course of the film) is more successful than a 'coping' model (in which the child is seen to be functioning well throughout, Burstein & Meichenbaum, 1979). Others have distinguished between the appropriateness of the models. Melamed & Siegel (1980) for example, have claimed that success is determined by the degree of perceived similarity between the child and model in terms of variables such as age, sex and race.

Few studies have, however, compared the differential effectiveness of films depending on qualitative differences in their content. One exception is a study by Zachary *et al.* (1985) who showed one of two films to children, aged between 3 and 11 years. The first was described as *stress-relevant* and showed a child coping adequately with painful dental treatment. The second was described as *stress-irrelevant* and showed a child coping adequately with having a plaster cast removed. Only the stress-relevant film was successful in reducing children's anxiety about dental treatment. Zachary *et al.* therefore argued that the content of the film is critical in determining how such films are received and interpreted by children.

In this fourth study, we are concerned particularly with the differential impact of the two films in the "Double Take" package. While both have the clear aim of educating and subsequently preventing drug abuse among children, the precise messages are quite different. In many ways, the "Minder" film has some of the elements of the modelling approach. Both 'coping' models and 'mastery' models are represented. At the same time, the film has considerable entertainment value. The "Thinking Twice" film is more clearly related to a 'life-skills/ decision-making' approach. In the study to be reported, pupils were divided into three groups; those who only viewed "Minder"; those who only viewed "Thinking Twice", and a control group who saw neither film. After viewing the film, pupils' attitudes and knowledge about drugs were assessed by questionnaire, and compared with responses given by the control group.

There were two other aims of this study. We were also interested in how the films were received by pupils depending on two variables: sex and previous experience. Previous research has shown that boys and girls differ in their experience of drugs and attitudes towards them (e.g., Yamaguchi & Kandell, 1984). In the research concerned with preparing children for hospitalization, Melamed & Siegel (1984) have shown that children's reactions to a film about hospital were determined by their history of previous hospital admissions. Although we did not attempt to collect data about pupils' experience with illicit drugs, we did collect self-report data about their experience with legal ones, particularly tobacco. There is some evidence that young people may 'progress' from experience with legal drugs to illegal ones (Kandell & Logan, 1984; Yamaguchi & Kandell, 1984). That is to say, although most who have taken legal drugs will not go on to take illegal ones, those who take illegal drugs will generally have taken legal ones first. We expected that sex and smoking status would affect pupils' attitudes to drugs, with boys and those who smoked being more knowledgeable and favourable towards drug abuse. As a practical concern, it is also valuable to determine if these variables predict pupils' ratings of the two films. Finally, we were concerned with the impact of the two films in different schools. The study involved pupils from seven comprehensives. The schools were drawn from the South West of England, and the Midlands, and included those from rural and more urban areas. One school catered for a predominantly black population.

Method

(a) *Subjects*

A total of 518 pupils were drawn from 7 mixed-sex comprehensive schools.

There was no systematic drugs education in any of the schools, and none of the pupils had seen the "Double Take" package before. Pupils were drawn from 3rd and 4th years (average age = 14 years). All pupils who were at school on the day we carried out the study and were in the selected classes took part.

Procedure

The procedure was the same in all schools. Pupils were divided into three approximately equal groups and the groups then randomly assigned to one of the three conditions. In the *experimental* conditions, pupils were told that they were to view a film about drug-taking and afterwards would be asked to complete a questionnaire to find out what they had learned and what their opinions were about the film. It was stressed that the film was in widespread use, and that their opinions were highly valued. If there was time after the questionnaires were completed, the pupils were encouraged to talk about their reactions to the film. These discussions were tape-recorded. Pupils in the *control* condition were asked to complete a questionnaire about drugs. It was emphasized that we were interested in their views and pupils were encouraged not to cheat or feel obliged to give the same responses as their neighbours. Pupils in the control condition were shown the "Minder" film after the questionnaires were completed. The number of pupils in each condition as a function of school is shown in Table 5.1.

Questionnaire

Pupils in the experimental condition were asked three questions to investigate their reactions to the film:-

'What did you think of the film you've just seen?'

'What did you think of the people in the film?'

'Did you learn anything from the film? If you did, please write it down'.

The rest of the questionnaire was the same for all groups, and consisted of many of the items described in previous chapters. The following items were included:-

(1) *Knowledge of drugs.*

(2) *Smoking and drinking habits, and amount of money available to spend.*

(3) *Self-ratings of school work.*

(4) *Perceptions of parental behaviour.*

(5) *Social competence.*

(6) *Attitudes to drug-taking.*

(7) *Perceptions of the addictive nature of substances.*

(8) *Beliefs about how to stop people taking drugs.*

TABLE 5.1

Sex distribution and number of pupils in each condition as a function of school

Sch.	*Region*	*Boys*	*Girls*	*Minder*	*T.T.*	*Control*	*Total*	*% of Sample*
A	Avon	38	31	29	22	25	69	13.3
B	Avon	47	33	19	34	27	80	15.4
C	Somerset	56	53	49	31	34	111	21.4
D	Birming.	30	23	17	22	19	58	11.2
E	Wiltsh.	37	37	25	24	28	77	14.9
F	Birming.	47	20	12	33	26	71	13.7
G	Bristol	22	26	23	15	14	52	10.7
			$\sum$	164	181	173	518	100

Results

Impact of the videos on attitude ratings

To investigate how the immediate impact of the films affected pupils' ratings of the addictiveness of drugs, their perceptions of why people take drugs and beliefs about how to stop them taking drugs, a series of multivariate analyses of variance were conducted. In the following analyses, sex and condition were used as 'between subjects' factors and ratings as a 'within subjects' factor. The analyses enabled us to compare ratings (1) across all three conditions (2) between the two experimental conditions and controls and (3) between "Minder" and "Thinking Twice".

Ratings of risk

The mean ratings of 'addictiveness' and 'likely to kill' for the 13 substances across the three experimental conditions are shown in Table 5.2. Overall, these ratings differed significantly across the three conditions ($F(52, 800) = 2.11$, $p < .001$). However, this effect was not due to differences between the two experimental *vs.* control conditions ($F(26, 399) = 1.07, ns$) but rather to differences in ratings between those who viewed "Minder" and those who viewed "Thinking Twice" ($F(26, 399) = 3.27$, $p < .001$).

A series of univariate F tests (each with df = 1,424) showed that significant differences between the two film conditions in ratings occurred on the following items:- Those who viewed "Thinking Twice" rated tea/coffee as more addictive ($F = 13.25$) and likely to kill ($F = 18.01$) than those who viewed "Minder". Those who viewed "Thinking Twice" also rated beer as more likely to kill ($F = 18.68$). All other significant differences were in the opposite direction, i.e. those who viewed "Minder" rated tranquillizers, heroin, spirits, glue, cocaine, LSD and cannabis as more addictive, and glue, cocaine, sleeping pills and LDS as more likely to kill than those who viewed "Thinking Twice".

Beliefs about persuasion

There was a significant difference on ratings of 'persuasion' depending on the experimental condition ($F(20, 916) = 2.42$, $p < .001$). Some of this difference could be accounted for by comparing the two groups who viewed the films with those in the control condition ($F(10, 457) = 2.04$, $p < .05$). However, there was also a significant difference in their ratings between those who viewed "Minder" and those who viewed "Thinking Twice" ($F(10, 457) = 2.79$, $p < .01$). A series of univariate F tests (with df = 1,466) showed that the main differences between the experimental groups

TABLE 5.2

Mean item ratings for addictiveness and likelihood of killing of the 13 substances

Item	Mean Scores			
	Minder	*T.T.*	*Control*	$F(1, 424)$
ADDICTIVENESS:				
Chocolate	3.11	3.43	2.78	1.69
Tranquillizers	5.81	5.24	5.28	7.23**
Tea or Coffee	3.82	4.70	3.89	13.25***
Cigarettes	6.68	6.53	6.55	1.52
Heroin	6.81	6.49	6.78	5.31*
Beer	5.75	5.78	5.84	0.03
Spirits	6.39	5.97	6.16	8.85**
Glue	6.69	6.23	6.52	9.67**
Cocaine	6.77	6.50	6.73	3.73*
Sleeping Pills	5.65	5.33	5.54	2.80
Vitamin Pills	4.07	4.31	4.11	1.04
LSD	6.37	5.96	6.18	4.85*
Cannabis	6.67	6.38	6.72	3.73*
LIKELY TO KILL:				
Chocolate	1.42	1.66	1.47	3.13
Tranquillizers	5.56	5.39	5.47	0.70
Tea or Coffee	1.64	2.41	2.12	18.01***
Cigarettes	6.56	6.53	6.43	0.09
Heroin	6.96	6.91	6.97	1.80
Beer	4.84	5.69	5.33	18.68***
Spirits	5.82	6.03	5.81	1.50
Glue	6.80	6.63	6.73	4.13*
Cocaine	6.93	6.84	6.95	3.88*
Sleeping Pills	5.99	5.78	5.74	4.72*
Vitamin Pills	3.30	3.61	3.51	1.83
LSD	6.61	6.32	6.30	5.08*
Cannabis	6.79	6.73	6.87	0.37

$***p < .001$ $**p < .01$ $*p < .05$

were in their ratings of the 'other drugs' items. Those who viewed "Thinking Twice" rated these items more positive than those who viewed "Minder". The mean ratings of all the items about persuasion are shown in Table 5.3.

TABLE 5.3

Mean item ratings for "Do you believe that in order to persuade young people not to take drugs like heroin it is a good idea to ... ":

	Mean Scores			
		Thinking		
Item	*Minder*	*Twice*	*Control*	$F(1,466)$
Make them scared	4.68	4.75	4.79	0.06
Talk about alcohol and tobacco	4.20	4.95	4.42	10.97***
Talk about tea and coffee	2.42	3.37	2.97	20.12***
Help them imagine being offered heroin	5.65	5.58	5.26	0.13
Help them say no	5.64	5.61	5.92	0.01
Talk about worries	5.61	5.57	5.85	0.04
Help them feel good	5.62	5.57	5.87	0.11
Help them make decisions	5.87	5.79	5.75	0.27
Give them information	6.43	6.44	6.42	0.01

$***p < .001$

Reasons why young people start taking drugs

Again, there were overall significant differences in ratings of these items by subjects in the three conditions ($F(40,878) = 2.60$, $p < .001$). These results were partly attributable to a difference between subjects who viewed either film and the control group ($F(20,438) = 1.68$, $p < .05$). The only individual item to distinguish between these groups however was 'They're given too much freedom' ($F(1,457) = 4.38, p < .04$). A comparison between those who viewed "Minder" and those who viewed "Thinking Twice" was also significant ($F(20,438) = 3.60$, $p < .001$). A series of univariate F

TABLE 5.4

Mean item ratings for "Why do young people start taking drugs?"

Item	Mean Scores Minder	Thinking Twice	Control	$F(1,457)$
Parents don't look after them	3.51	3.92	3.47	3.94*
Want to try something new	5.48	5.32	5.18	0.81
Don't think of consequences	5.61	5.17	5.35	4.61*
Problems at school	4.14	4.78	4.34	2.94
Given too much freedom	3.88	4.08	3.57	0.71
Pushed by others	6.33	5.87	6.26	9.07**
Problems at home	4.94	5.10	4.91	0.66
No sense of right or wrong	4.28	4.22	3.99	0.07
Bad company	6.34	6.03	5.95	4.41*
Think it will be fun	6.14	5.72	5.67	6.01**
Only once	6.56	6.20	6.15	7.30**
Wrong place	4.39	4.45	4.54	0.09
Feel low	4.91	4.93	5.07	0.01
Too much publicity	3.20	3.45	3.64	1.27
Bored	4.20	4.53	4.04	2.13
Exciting to take risks	5.02	5.09	4.97	0.10
See adults drinking	4.77	5.44	4.98	9.99**
Want to look grown up	5.41	6.25	5.57	20.89***
Won't get a job	3.65	3.91	3.87	1.41
Get hold of drugs easily	5.14	5.15	5.23	0.00

$***p < .001$ $\quad **p < .01$ $\quad *p < .05$

tests (with df = 1,457) revealed a number of items which distinguished between these two groups. Items which were rated more positively by those who viewed "Minder" included 'They don't think about the consequences', 'They're pushed into it by others', 'They get into bad company', and 'They think it will be only once'. Items which were rated more positively by those who viewed "Thinking Twice" included 'Their parents don't look after them properly', 'They see adults drinking, and smoking', and 'They want to look grown up'. These data are summarized in Table 5.4.

Social Competence

A multivariate analysis of variance on these data revealed no significant differences related to experimental conditions (see Table 5.5).

TABLE 5.5

Mean item rating on the Social Competence scale

	Means		
Item	Minder	Thinking Twice	Control
Get on with people your age	5.87	5.71	5.85
Get on with people you don't know	4.80	4.60	4.70
Get on in new places	4.60	4.77	4.66
Get on with adults	5.29	5.21	5.36
Get on with parents	5.81	6.01	6.11
Get on with teachers	4.67	4.96	4.62
Understand others' feelings	5.25	5.20	5.16
Make decisions	5.76	5.80	5.70
Say "no"	6.01	5.82	5.63
Cheer yourself up	4.91	4.89	4.67

Relationships with parents

There was no significant effect of condition on pupils' ratings of their relationships with parents.

(b) *Impact of the videos as a function of pupils' sex*

Ratings of risk

Boys and girls differed significantly in rating the addictiveness and dangerousness of substances ($F(26, 399) = 1.92$, $p < .01$). However, there was no Sex x Condition interaction ($F(52, 800) = 0.96, ns$) showing that the impact of the two videos was not confounded by pupils' sex.

Beliefs about persuasion

Again, there was a significant main effect for Sex ($F(10, 457) = 2.84$, $p < .002$), without a significant Sex x Condition interaction ($F(20, 916) = 1.07, ns$). The sex effect was largely attributable to ratings on four items. Girls agreed more with the following items than boys:- 'Talk about medicines at the same time as heroin', 'Help them to imagine being offered heroin', 'Help them to talk about personal problems and worries', 'Help them to feel good about themselves'.

Reasons why young people start taking drugs

Again, despite a significant main effect of Sex ($F(20, 438) = 2.34$, $p < .001$), there was no Sex x Condition interaction ($F(40, 878) = 1.04, ns$). The Sex effect was due primarily to girls agreeing with the following statements: 'They don't think about the consequences', 'They're having problems at school', 'They're pushed into it by other young people', 'They think it will be fun', 'They tell themselves it will only be once', 'They want to look grown up'.

Social competence

These results follow a similar pattern; a significant Sex effect ($F(10, 472) = 6.67$, $p < .001$), due largely to girls agreeing more with the following items: 'Get on with people you don't know', 'Get on in new places', 'Get on with adults', 'Understand others' feelings', and 'Say no'. Again there was no sex by condition interaction ($F(20, 946) = 0.72, ns$).

Relationships with parents

Again, there was a significant main effect for Sex ($F(8,457) = 3.81$, $p < .001$). Girls agreed more with two statements 'my parents always know where I am' and 'my parents treat me like a baby'. There was no Sex x Condition interaction ($F(16, 916) = 1.56, ns$).

(c) *Impact of the videos as a function of smoking status*

A subsidiary set of multivariate analyses of variance were conducted, using current smoking status and condition as 'between subject' factors, and ratings as a 'within subjects' factor. Subjects were divided into three groups depending on their smoking status: those who claimed they had never smoked; those who had smoked but had given up, and those who were regular smokers.

Beliefs about persuasion

There was a main effect of Smoking status on ratings of these items ($F(20, 918) = 1.67$, $p < .03$). In particular, there was a significant effect on ratings on one item ('help them to imagine being offered heroin'). Those who had never smoked agreed least with this item (mean = 5.51), compared with those who used to smoke (mean = 6.12). However, there was no smoking status by condition effect ($F(40, 1848) = 1.06, ns$).

Reasons why young people start taking drugs

Again, there was a main effect for current Smoking status ($F(40, 882) = 1.68$, $p < .01$). The Condition x Smoking status interaction ($F(80, 1772) = 1.34$, $p < .05$) was also significant.

Social competence

Ratings of these items were affected by Smoking status ($F(20, 956) = 2.83$, $p < .001$). A series of univariate F tests (with df = 2,486) showed that current smokers, those who had given up and those who had never tried differed especially in their ratings of the following items, 'Get on with your parents', 'Get on with your teachers' and 'Say 'no' when you feel you shouldn't do something'. However, there was no Condition x Smoker status interaction, ($F(40, 1920) = 1.11$).

Relationships with parents

Again, there was a main effect of Smoker status ($F(16, 930) = 3.45$, $p < .001$). Univariate F tests showed that ratings between the smoker status groups were particularly significant, as follows. Those who had never smoked were more likely to endorse the statements 'My parents always know where I am and what I'm doing', 'My parents are more strict than most parents', and 'My parents still treat me like a baby'. Those who were current smokers were more likely than non-smokers to endorse 'I decide things for myself even when my parents disagree with me'. However, there was no Condition x Smoker status interaction ($F(32, 1868) = 0.72$).

(d) *Impact of the videos as a function of school*

We first conducted a series of tests to look at differences between schools in terms of incidence of smoking and drinking behaviour, pupils' perceptions of their school work, and how much they had to spend. There were significant differences between the schools in terms of smoking habits ($\chi^2(36) = 54.80$, $p < .02$) whether pupils reported ever being really drunk (χ^2 $(12) = 41.77$, $p < .001$), their ratings of their own school work ($\chi^2(36) = 79.67$, $p < .001$) and how much they had to spend ($\chi^2(60) = 86.72$, $p < .01$).

In order to investigate whether these school differences were reflected in pupils' ratings of attitudes to drugs, a series of multivariate analyses of variance were then conducted, using school and condition as 'between subjects' factors and ratings as 'within subjects'.

Ratings of risk

As shown in the previous analyses, there was a main effect for Condition ($F(52, 794) = 2.15$, $p < .001$). In addition, ratings were affected by School ($F(156, 2406) = 1.51$, $p < .001$) and there was a significant Condition x School interaction ($F(312, 4884) = 1.31$, $p < .001$).

Beliefs about persuasion

Ratings of these items were significantly affected by School ($F(60, 2760)$ $= 1.51$, $p < .01$). A series of univariate F tests showed that these differences were particularly reflected in two items. These were 'Help them to feel good about themselves', and 'Help them to make decisions for themselves'. In addition, there was a significant Condition x School interaction, ($F(120, 4640) = 1.46$, $p < .001$). A series of univariate F tests revealed the following significant differences Talk about tea and coffee at the same time as heroin', 'Talk about medicines at the same time as heroin', 'Help them to practice saying no', and 'Give them as much information as possible'.

Reasons why young people start taking drugs

Again, there was a main effect for School ($F(120, 2652) = 1.72$, $p <$ $.001$) showing that beliefs about why people start to take drugs varied from school to school. A series of univariate F tests showed that these differences were most pronounced on the following items: 'Their parents don't look after them properly', 'They're pushed into it by other young people', 'They tell themselves it will only be once', 'There's too much publicity about drugs', 'They're bored', 'They see adults drinking and smoking', and 'They want to look grown up'. Despite these differences, the Condition x School interaction was not significant, ($F(240, 5376) = 1.14, ns$).

Social competence

Again, there was a significant effect of School ($F(60, 2874) = 1.61$, $p < .01$), but a series of univariate F tests showed that this was primarily due to two items. These were 'Get on with teachers', and 'Say no when you feel you shouldn't do something'. The Condition x School interaction was not significant, ($F(120, 4830) = 1.15, ns$).

Relationships with parents

On these items there were no significant effects due to Achool ($F(48, 2784) = 1.09$) or Condition x School interaction, ($F(96, 3728) = 1.12$).

(e) *Qualitative analyses*

The open-ended questions concerned with pupils' evaluations of the videos and knowledge of drugs were coded by two independent raters. The frequencies of particular categories of response were then compared between conditions.

Evaluation of the films

These data are summarized in Table 5.6. A χ^2 test on these data was significant ($\chi^2(6) = 16.74$, $p < .02$). This result was due to the fact that more pupils rated "Minder" to be of positive entertainment value than did those who watched "Thinking Twice". However, slightly more pupils rated "Thinking Twice" to be of positive educational value than those who watched "Minder". Only 11 pupils expessed the view that the films should be made more 'scary'; 4 who saw "Minder" and 7 who saw "Thinking Twice".

TABLE 5.6

Pupils' evaluation of Minder and Thinking Twice

Film	*Entert.*		*Educat.*	
	Positive	Negative	Positive	Negative
Minder	51.5	3.0	17.9	6.0
T. T.	36.2	10.9	26.1	5.8
	+ Ent + Ed	+ Ent - Ed	- Ent + ED	- Ent - Ed
Minder	14.9	5.2	1.5	0
T. T.	16.7	1.4	1.4	1.4

Evaluation of the people in the films

Again, there were differences in the way that pupils rated the people in the two films. These data are summarized in Table 5.7. More pupils rated the people in "Thinking Twice" unfavourably. At the same time, pupils who saw "Minder" were more likely than those who watched "Thinking Twice" to express mixed feelings about the characters ($\chi^2(2) = 21.31, p < .001$).

TABLE 5.7

Pupils' evaluations of the people in the films

	Ratings		
	Positive	*Negative*	*Mixed*
"Minder"	68.0	9.4	22.7
"Thinking Twice"	61.9	29.1	9.0

Pupils' reports about what they learned from the films

These data are summarized in Table 5.8. Although the frequencies of pupils in any category are relatively small, there are some differences in expected directions. Those who saw "Thinking Twice" were more likely to report learning the names of drugs than those who saw "Minder"($\chi^2(1) =$ 5.22, $p < .02$. They also were more likely to report that they learned how 'common' drugs were, referring particularly to caffeine in tea, coffee and soft drinks ($\chi^2(1) = 17.93$, $p < .001$). Conversely, pupils who viewed

"Minder" were more likely than those who viewed "Thinking Twice" to mention that they learned about the adverse social consequences of taking drugs ($\chi^2(1) = 17.35$, $p < .001$).

TABLE 5.8

Pupils' reports about what they learned from the films

	"Minder"	"Thinking Twice"
Names	1.4	7.8
Addiction	16.5	10.5
Commonness	0.7	15.0
Saying "no"	15.8	12.4
Stealing	13.7	0.7
Decisions	0.7	3.3
Availability	1.4	0.7

Knowledge items

More pupils in the "Thinking Twice" condition gave reasonably accurate descriptions of a 'stimulant' than pupils in the "Minder" or control conditions ($\chi^2(6) = 25.79$, $p < .001$). However, there were no differences between the three conditions in terms of the number of stimulant drugs that pupils could name, ($\chi^2(8) = 12.25, ns$). Similarly, pupils in the "Thinking Twice" condition were more likely to give reasonable accounts of the meaning of 'tolerance' than pupils in the other two conditions (χ^2 (6) $= 30.34$, $p < .001$), as well as understand that the danger of injecting drugs rather than taking them by mouth was due to the speed with which drugs could then circulate round the blood-system ($\chi^2(12) = 43.67$, $p < .001$. Pupils who saw "Thinking Twice" were also more likely to be aware that the brain and nervous system were particularly at risk if drugs were taken ($\chi^2(8) = 22.30$, $p < .01$. There were no other significant differences between the three conditions.

Discussion

Despite the fact that "Double Take" was intended to be integrated within a social/health education programme and was produced along with suggested teaching activities and exercises, there has always been concern that the films would be used without follow-up work, and particularly to cover staff absences or 'wet playtimes'. This concern might be especially relevant in the case of "Minder", given its more entertaining appeal. As reported in Chapter 2, those teachers who responded to our questionnaire did not indicate that this happened frequently. Even so, the results of this study are particularly relevant to situations where pupils are shown either video, and no attempt at follow-up work is made. We also feel that the results are relevant to situations where pupils are involved with a programme based exclusively on "Minder" or "Thinking Twice". Our data suggest that the impacts of the two videos are different; whether these differences are enhanced or reduced by appropriate follow-up work requires additional research.

It seems to us that, at a general level, "Minder" is more successful than "Thinking Twice" in promoting more negative attitudes towards drugs. This is based on the finding that, after viewing "Minder", pupils shifted their ratings of the addictiveness and dangerousness of a number of substances in the direction of greater rejection. For those who viewed "Thinking Twice" the shift was only on two items. Specifically, these pupils rated tea and coffee as more addictive and dangerous after seeing the film, and beer as more dangerous. Their ratings of other substances tended to be in the opposite direction. The effect of "Thinking Twice" appears to be that pupils differentiate less between substances. One of the main messages of "Thinking Twice" is that pupils can learn from their experiences with legal drugs as to how they might handle situations in which they were offered illegal ones. With this aim in mind, the perception of similarities between legal and illegal drugs might be regarded as a success.

We also found shifts in pupils' ratings of items concerned with why people start to take drugs which were specific to the two videos. After viewing "Minder", pupils tended to agree more with items concerned with not thinking about the consequences, being pushed by others, getting into bad company and thinking it will be only once. All these reflect issues that are central to the film. In the party scene, the principal character comes under pressure from peers to take drugs, and suggestions are voiced that it need only be for once. In contrast, those who viewed "Thinking Twice" agreed more with items implicating lack of parental control, and wanting to look 'grown-up' or follow adult examples in drinking and smoking. The message in "Thinking Twice" is much less concerned with peer pressure or taking drugs for 'fun'. It is much more concerned with encouraging pupils to observe adult behaviour and subsequently make informed decisions about which drugs, if any, they wish to take.

Similar arguments can be made about pupils' responses to items concerned with their beliefs about the best way to stop people taking drugs. As might be expected, pupils who viewed "Thinking Twice" tended to endorse items concerned with talking about heroin together with other drugs more than those who viewed "Minder". It is not clear why there were no significant differences on any of the other items. As hypothesized in the previous chapter, it may be that pupils find the decision-making approach difficult, given that it is not the usual method of teaching in school. Once again, it seems to us that one of the main limitations of this package is that it stands alone. Pupils are confronted with a style of teaching and an approach that are distinct from much of their previous experience. There would appear to be arguments for adopting a similar approach to teaching at least in other areas of health and social education, even if not in more traditional subjects.

Despite differences in sex, smoking status and school of pupils who took part in this study, there were few systematic effects as a function of these variables on attitudes which were specific to either film. This must be seen as a very heartening result. Many teachers have expressed concerns that the videos might not have general appeal. Particular criticisms of "Minder" have included the under-representation of female characters, black characters and the fact that it is clearly set in South London. These objections are less valid for "Thinking Twice". Nevertheless, pupils do not seem to rate either video very differently as a function of sex, smoking status or school, suggesting that the films do have a degree of general appeal.

6

The impact of "Double Take" as a function of region and extent of use

Introduction

Evaluations of decision-making approaches to drugs education have predominantly been conducted in white, middle-class schools in the United States, (Battjes & Bell, 1985). This is a serious shortcoming, since it is not clear how well the approach may be acceptable to pupils from deprived or ethnic backgrounds. One of the aims of this final study is to assess any differential impact of "Double Take" in different parts of England (excluding Wales and Scotland).

A second aim was to investigate how pupils' attitudes to drugs were affected by the way in which "Double Take" was used. It is recommended in the teachers' notes that follow-up work is an essential part of the package, the assumption being that this is necessary for pupils to derive maximum benefit from the videos. Yet it is also clear that many teachers are unable or unwilling to devote much curriculum time to such follow-up work. We therefore attempted to compare attitudes among pupils who had experienced relatively extensive follow-up work (approximately 6 hours including time to see the video) with attitudes among those who had experienced very little follow-up work (approximately 1 hour including time to see the video).

Method

(a) *Subjects*

Schools were selected for this study on the basis of teachers' responses to the postal questionnaire (study 1). Since the results of this study showed that a majority of secondary schools concentrated their drugs education on 4th year pupils, we based our selection of 'high' and 'low' user schools on teachers' reports of how extensively "Double Take" was used with 4th year pupils. We used responses to the question 'How many hours are devoted to drugs education generally and "Double Take" specifically both in the academic years 1985-1986 and 1986-1987?'. In fact, teachers' responses to this question were highly skewed, perhaps due to a reluctance to make quantitative judgements of this kind, but also because schools do not seem to have a general policy, so that the amount of curriculum time devoted to drugs education may be variable, depending on particular teachers' interests.

On this basis, however, we identified 12 likely 'high' user schools who had reported that they assigned 6 or more curriculum hours to the package. These were distributed geographically from the North West to the South East. A further 8 'low' user schools from the same regions were also approached. These 'low' user schools indicated that they assigned very little or no curriculum time to teaching based on "Double Take".

Despite the fact that all these schools had indicated their willingness to be involved in further research, and although repeated attempts were made to contact relevant teachers, the schools, especially the 'low' users, were slow to respond. The final sample consisted of 6 'high' user and 1 'low' user school. (Two other schools agreed to take part the following term). The 'high' user schools were in Barrow-in-Furness, Preston, Shrewsbury, Worcester, Sutton Coldfield and Norwich and the 'low' user school was in Birmingham. In all schools, the sample consisted of 3-4 classes of 4th year pupils and 1-2 classes of 2nd year pupils.

(b) *Questionnaire*

The questionnaire included many of the items described in previous studies.

We included one additional section which had not been used previously (see Appendix B). This consisted of ten items, each to be rated on a 7 point scale from 'strongly disagree' to 'strongly agree'. Some of these items were based partly on a previous study by Eiser and Gossop (1979), which attempted to distinguish ways in which drug-use could be seen as an addiction and/or sickness.

In addition, we asked pupils to estimate the amount and type of teaching about drugs that they remembered. First, they were given a list of 11 films about drugs, and asked to tick any that they had seen. Second, they were asked to estimate how many lessons (none, 1-3, 4-9, 10 or more) about drugs which they remembered for different parts of the curriculum (biology, health/social education, tutor groups, religion or 'other' lessons). They were then asked if they remembered any lessons at all concerned with various aspects of drugs and drug-taking (heroin, glue) solvent sniffing, cannabis, cigarettes, alcohol, cocaine, other drugs, drug-taking and AIDS, advertising).

(c) *Procedure*

Schools were first contacted by letter. If the school replied, we then telephoned to describe the study in more detail and arrange how the questionnaires were to be distributed. Schools who did not respond were contacted again by letter and telephone. In five of the seven schools, we arranged to visit and distribute the questionnaires. In the remaining two, teachers preferred to distribute the questionnaires themselves.

(d) *Design*

The fact that we had only one 'low' user school precluded the possibility of looking for *interactive* effects of region and level of use. However, this weakness in the sample was off-set by two other considerations. First, the inclusion of 2nd- year pupils (with whom the package had not been used at all) provided a form of control group within each school. Although not ideal, this should still provide some indication of effects due to catchment area. Second, the greater part of the questionnaire was identical with that used in the previous study, in which pupils were shown either "Minder" or "Thinking Twice" or assigned to a 'no-film' control group. All the schools in this previous study would have qualified as 'low' users. The control group of this previous study could thus be combined with the single 'low' user school for most of the relevant statistical analyses. (In fact, when the older age group from the 'low user' school was compared with the combined control groups from the previous study, no systematic differences were found).

Thus, there were two complementary designs: (1) A design consisting of 7 schools (6 'high' users and 1 'low' user) with two age- groups in each school; (2) A design, based on 14 schools (though excluding the younger age-group from the present sample and the two 'experimental' groups from the previous sample) combined to form a single 'high' user and a single 'low' user group. Design (1) is better suited to the detection of regional and age differences, while design (2) provides a simpler and more reliable indicator of differences attributable to the extent of use of the package.

Results

1. *Analyses of differences between the seven schools.*

A series of multivariate analyses of variance were conducted, including as factors sex, age-group and school. Table 6.1 shows the number of pupils in each cell of the design. The school factor was partitioned into six orthogonal contrasts. The first contrast compared the six high user schools with the one low user school, the remainder involving comparisons between the different high users.

TABLE 6.1

Number of pupils included from each school.

Age group	Young	(2nd Year)	Old	4th Year
Sex	M	F	M	F
Barrow-in-Furness	12	13	16	12
Sutton Coldfield	11	11	104	93
Preston	13	17	28	25
Worcester	7	16	86	75
Shewsbury	8	11	32	38
Norfolk	16	12	39	47
Birmingham (lower user)	12	8	21	31
Total	79	88	326	321

(a) *Perceptions of parental behaviour*

There were significant multivariate effects for Sex ($F(8,753) = 5.05, p < .001$), Age-group ($F(8,753) = 6.61, p < .001$) and School ($F(48,4548) = 1.87, p < .001$), and the Age-group x School interaction ($F(48,4548) =$

$1.47, p < .05$). All the other effects were nonsignificant, although the Age-group x Sex interaction was marginal ($F(8, 173) = 1.90, p < .06$). Univariate tests (with df = 1,780) revealed that the Sex effect depended mainly on three items: 'My parents keep changing their minds about what I can and cannot do' (means: boys, 2.58, girls, 2.36; $F = 18.27, p < .001$), 'My parents always know where I am and what I'm doing' (means: 3.47, 3.87; $F = 11.09, p < .001$) and 'My parents are more strict than most parents' (means: 2.49, 2.33; $F = 4.35, p < .05$). The Age-group effect depended on the second of the above items (means: young, 4.08, old, 3.57; $F = 27.32, p < .001$), as well as on 'I decide things for myself even when my parents disagree with me' (means: 2.52, 3.03; $F = 27.40, p < .001$).

The main effect of School and the School x Age-group interaction were investigated further by analyses within each age-group. The first contrast of the School effect (high vs. low user) was significant for the older but not the younger age group. Among the older pupils, those in the low user school saw their parents as 'changing their minds' more often ($F(1, 612) = 7.11, p < .01$) but also as knowing their whereabouts to a greater extent ($F(1, 612) = 11.84, p < .001$). There was a tendency for an 'East-West' regional difference (Norfolk and Sutton-Coldfield vs. Worcester and Shrewsbury) in the older groups, but not in the younger group, among whom the main regional difference was between the two Northern schools (Preston and Barrow) and the other four high users.

(b) *Ratings of dangerousness of different substances*

For these items, two within-subjects factors were incorporated in the design: Addictive vs. Kill ratings, and Substance. Among the most noteworthy effects, there was a large effect for Substance ($F(12, 686) = 321.91$; $p <$ 001) reflecting the fact that some substances were rated as more dangerous than others, interactions between Substance and Addictive vs. Kill ($F(12, 686) = 40.58; p < .001$), Sex ($F(12, 686) = 3.59, p < .001$); Age-group ($F(12, 686) = 2.39, p < .01$) and School ($F(72, 4146) = 2.02, p < .001$).

The Addictive vs. Kill effect was significant overall ($F(1, 697) = 41.82$, $p < .001$) reflecting the fact that the substances were seen as more addictive than lethal. This factor interacted significantly with Age-group ($F(1, 697) =$

$9.78, p < .01$) and School ($F(6,697) = 5.18, p < .001$) but not Sex ($F(1,697) = 3.38$, $p < .07$). There were main effects for Age-group ($F(1,697) = 6.17, p < .05$) and School ($F(6,697) = 7.73, p < .001$), these two factors interacting significantly ($F(6,697) = 3.72, p < .001$).

Additional analyses (without the within subjects factors) indicated that, among the older, but not the younger subjects, the contrast between the low user school and the remaining six was significant ($F(26,546) = 2.13, p < .001$). This reflected the fact that the low user school gave the lowest mean ratings of the addictiveness of tea/coffee, beer, spirits and sleeping pills (means respectively: 3.07, 5.35. 5.80, 4.96; Univariate $Fs(1,571) = 26.87, p < .001; 4.39, p < .05; 8.17, p < .01; 7.28, p < .01$) and of the lethality of tea/coffee, beer and spirits (means: 1.85, 4.60, 5.34, $Fs(1,571) = 4.41, p < .05; 7.02, p < .01; 10.54, p < .001$). There were numerous differences among the high user schools but these did not suggest a clear regional pattern. Among the younger subjects, these differences were less.

(c) *Reasons why young people start taking drugs*

There were significant multivariate effects for Sex ($F(20,696) = 2.55$, $p < .001$), Age-group ($F(20,696) = 2.75, p < .001$) and School ($F(120, 4206) = 2.03$, $p < .001$), but no interactions. Univariate tests (with df = 1,715) showed that the Sex differences were most marked in terms of attributions to lack of parental care (means: boys, 3.93, girls, 3.47, $F = 7.72, p < .01$), pressure from other young people (means, 6.01, 6.26; $F = 5.45, p < .05$), too much freedom (means, 4.17, 3.98; $F = 5.29, p < .05$) being in the wrong place at the wrong time (means, 4.67, 4.84; $F = 4.94, p < .05$) and job worries (means, 3.93, 3.75; $F = 4.09, p < .05$). The Age-group differences were most marked on lack of parental care (means: young, 4.12, old, 3.58; $F = 14.96, p < .001$), no sense of right and wrong (means, 4.75, 4.18; $F = 11.51, p < .001$), adult example (means, 5.38, 4.70; $F = 7.67, p < .01$), publicity (means, 4.11, 3.52; $F = 5.73, p < .05$), too much freedom (means, 4.38, 3.99: $F = 4.95, p < .05$) and a wish to look grown up (means, 5.91, 5.56; $F = 4.38, p < .05$).

With regard to the School effect, the contrast between the six high users and the single low user school was significant ($F(20,696) = 3.65, p <$

.001) as was the same contrast within the Age-group x School interaction ($F(20, 696) = 1.65, p < .05$). When the two Age-groups are considered separately, the contrast is significant for the older ($F(20, 562) = 2.64, p < .001$) but not the younger ($F(20, 115) = 1.02, ns$) group. Univariate tests showed that, with the older group, the low user school was the least likely of the seven schools to explain drug-use in terms of being in the wrong place, finding risks exciting, job worries, availability of drugs, too much freedom, and no sense of right and wrong (means respectively: 3.98, 4.41, 3.04, 4.48, 3.37, 3.63; Univariate $Fs(1, 581) = 9.13, p < .01; 8.94, p < .01; 8.26, p < .01; 6.96, p < .01; 4.85, p < .05; 4.43, p < .05$). As with other items, there were various other significant differences between the schools which were more marked for older than younger subjects, but which did not suggest any simple pattern of regional differences.

(d) *Social competence*

Significant multivariate effects were obtained for Sex ($F(10, 739) = 4.34, p < .001$), Age-group ($F(10, 739) = 4.07, p < .01$), School ($F(60,4464) = 1.56, p < .01$), and the following interactions: Sex x Age-group ($F(10,739) = 2.23, p < .05$), Age-group x School ($F(60, 4464) = 1.52, p < .01$) and Sex x Age-group x School ($F(60, 4464) = 1.46, p < .05$). However, none of the effects relating to School are of great interest. The high vs. low user contrast was not significant overall, within each age group separately and as part of the interaction. Other differences between schools were unsystematic, and not constant over the two age groups. Univariate tests (with df = 1,748) indicated that the Sex effect was largely due to one item, the ability to understand other peoples' feelings, on which girls scored much higher (means: boys, 4.89, girls, 5.69; $F = 34.49, p < .001$), although girls scored somewhat higher than boys on most of the items, and significantly so on getting on with teachers (means, 4.57, 5.12; $F = 5.31, p < .05$). Older pupils felt more competent at making decisions for themselves (means: young 5.09, old 5.69; $F = 24.07, p < .001$), but got on less well with teachers (means, 5.28, 4.73, $F = 6.71, p < .01$) and parents (means, 6.21, 5.90; $F = 5.50, p < .05$).

(e) *Beliefs about persuasion*

The following significant multivariate effects were obtained: Sex (F(10,

727) = 3.67, $p < .001$), Age-group ($F(10,717) = 3.57, p < .001$), School ($F(60,4392) = 2.05, p < .001$); Age-group x School ($F(60,4392) = 1.62, p < .01$). The high vs. low user contrast is non-significant overall, although it approaches significance as part of the Age-group x School effect, and in the older group considered separately. The low user school gave the *lowest* endorsement to a scare approach (mean, 4.30; $F(1,606) = 8.51, p < .01$). Otherwise the school differences suggested no systematic pattern.

Six items showed significant effects of Sex by univariate tests (df = 1,736): help them talk about problems (means: boys, 5.52, girls, 6.16; $F = 17.66, p < .001$); help them to feel good about themselves (means, 5.50, 5.98; $F = 13.27, p < .001$), help them imagine being offered heroin (means, 4.72, 5.25; $F = 11.71, p < .001$) help them make decisions for themselves (means, 5.63, 5.91; $F = 9.49, p < .01$), give as much information as possible (means, 6.19,6.37; $F = 5.41, p < .05$) and talk about tea/coffee (means, 2.73, 2.89; $F = 4.09, p < .05$). The Age-group difference depended on two items: help them make decisions for themselves (means: young, 5.32, old, 5.88; $F = 14.42, p < .001$) and help them talk about problems (means, 5.99, 5.81; $F = 4.11, p < .05$).

(f) *Most suitable person to teach about drugs*

For this analysis, the design included one within-subjects factor – the six target persons being rated. There was a highly significant overall difference between the target persons ($F(5,742) = 82.03, p < .001$) but few other effects of note. These differences were mediated by Age-group ($F(5,742) = 3.90, p < .01$) but not by Sex or School. The Age-group main effect was also significant ($F(1,746) = 6.66, p < .01$). There were no other significant between-subjects effects, and a few more complex interactions involving the target person difference may safely be ignored. Table 6.2 shows the means for each Age-group and the univariate F ratios for the Age-group effect. As may be seen, the older pupils rated the suitability of an ex-drug addict higher, but that of all other target persons lower, than did younger pupils.

(g) *Beliefs about drug-use*

These 10 items, introduced for the first time in this study, were submitted to a similar analysis. There were significant multivariate effects for Sex ($F(10,686) = 1.86, p < .05$), Age-group ($F(10,686) = 2.90, p < .001$) and

School ($F(60, 4146) = 2.49, p < .001$). Univariate tests (with df = 1,695) indicated that girls were somewhat more likely to see drug-takers as 'just like other people' (means: boys, 3.85, girls, 4.32; $F = 4.96, p < .05$) and to believe it was difficult to stop taking drugs (means, 5.87, 6.21; $F = 4.20, p < .001$). The strongest age difference was on the item 'Drugs can really make you feel good' (means: young, 2.27, old, 3.21: $F = 17.53, p < .001$). There were also significant univariate age differences with regard to seeing a risk of AIDS (means, 4.75, 5.22; $F = 4.96, p < .05$) and believing that 'You can take drugs for fun without getting hooked' (means, 1.76, 2.16; $F = 4.44, p < .05$). The effect of School did not represent a significant high vs. low user difference. There were various differences among the high user schools. For example, the two more northerly schools seemed to be more inclined to regard drug-use as a sickness, and as difficult to stop, and to believe that drug-takers were terrified of withdrawal.

TABLE 6.2

Ratings of suitability to teach young people about drugs.

	Age group		F (1,746)	Overall mean
Person	Young	Old		
Parent	4.98	4.36	10.07**	4.48
Ex-drug addict	6.02	6.38	7.20**	6.32
Teacher	4.89	4.48	5.76*	4.45
Policeman	4.64	4.31	3.09	4.39
Doctor	6.03	5.77	3.01	5.89
Nurse	5.65	5.29	4.92*	5.41
N	149	625		774

$*p < .05$, $**p < .01$

(h) *Recall of drug education*

The first item measuring recall asked pupils to indicate any 'films about drugs and drug taking' that they remembered seeing, from a list of 11. The overall percentages for recall of each film were as follows: "Gail is dead", 12.5, "Minder", 72.1 "Chase the bandwagon", 3.8; "It's your life", 17.2;

"Free to choose", 3.1; "Better dead", 3.8; "Just say no", 73.5; "Grange Hill", 93.2; "BBC Drugwatch", 78.0; "Thinking Twice", 13.4; "Drugs and the Nervous System", 6.0. The corresponding percentages for the single low user school (Birmingham) were, respectively: 1.3, 64.5, 2.6, 27.6, 3.9, 5.3, 77.6, 94.7, 77.6, 2.6, 6.6.

The second item asked pupils to recall how many lessons (since the previous September) they had had about drugs and drug-taking in the following classes: biology/science, health/social education, tutor groups, religious education, and 'other'. Responses were in terms of the categories: no lessons, 1-3, 4-9 and 10 or more lessons. The percentages of the total sample recalling *any* lessons about drugs in each class were: biology/science, 26.5; health/social education, 45.1; tutor groups, 23.6; religious education, 39.7; other, 32.1. The corresponding figures for the Birmingham school were 12.7, 60.9, 30.6, 43.7 and 33.3.

The third recall question asked pupils to remember the topics covered in such lessons. The overall percentages recalling each topic were: heroin, 61.7; glue/solvent sniffing, 43.2; cannabis, 46.2; cigarettes, 82.1; alcohol, 74.0; cocaine, 48.0; any other drugs, 50.6; AIDS, 56.4; advertising of cigarettes/alcohol, 50.5. The corresponding percentages for the Birmingham school were generally below average: 46.5, 25.7, 10.0, 64.4, 62.5, 17.4, 22.1, 77.8 and 32.4. The interesting exception is that the percentage of pupils at Birmingham recalling a lesson about drug-taking and AIDS was the highest of the seven schools. It is also worth noting that recall of a lesson on AIDS was only weakly correlated with recall of the other eight topics, which intercorrelated quite highly (yielding a Cronbach's alpha of .829).

Interesting also are the results for the Preston school which had the strongest bias towards a biology/science as opposed to a social education approach (as judged from pupils' recall of numbers of lessons about drugs in different classes). The recall of lessons on specific topics by pupils from this school were consistently low: (respectively, 18.5, 18.5, 12.3, 56.1, 44.4, 13.6, 16.3, 40.7 and 34.6). Thus, although this school was a 'high user' in terms of the use of "Double Take" (as declared on the teachers' questionnaire), the pupils themselves seem not to have felt that they had had much teaching on specific drug-related topics.

2. *Analyses comparing combined samples of 'low', and 'high user' schools*

These analyses consisted of a series of multivariate analyses of variance with a simple 2 x 2 (Sex x School group) between-subjects design. The sample included 118 boys and 102 girls in the low user group and 305 boys and 290 girls in the high user group.

(a) *Perceptions of parental behaviour*

The multivariate tests revealed no significant differences due to Sex ($F(6,777) = 2.08, p < .06$), School group ($F(6,777) = 1.34$) or the interaction ($F(6,777) = 1.41$).

(b) *Ratings of dangerousness of different substances.*

These ratings were analysed with a more complex design incorporating two within-subjects factors: Addictive vs. Kill ratings and Substance. Table 6.3 shows the means for the low and high user schools. As these show, there were large differences between substances ($F(12,711) = 563.33, p < .001$). The ratings of addictiveness were rather higher than the lethality ratings ($F(1,722) = 108.22, p < .001$), and the interaction between the within-subjects factors was significant ($F(12,711) = 45.93, p < .001$). None of the between-subjects effects or interactions were significant, but there were there a number of significant interactions between the between- and within-subjects factors. Sex interacted significantly with Addictive vs. Kill ($F(1,722) = 14.52, p < .001$), with Substance ($F(12,711) = 3.35, p < .001$), but not with their interaction. School-group interacted with Addictive vs. Kill ($F(1,722) = 5.05, p < .05$), Substance ($F(12,711) = 4.12, p < .001$) and their interaction ($F(12,711) = 1.87, p < .05$). These effects reflected the fact that the distinction between ratings of addictiveness and lethality was clearer for girls than boys, and for those in the high rather than low user schools. Girls rated tranquillizers ($F(1,722) = 14.52, p < .001$) and glue ($F(1,722) = 16.65, p < .001$) as more addictive, and LSD as less addictive ($F(1,722) = 11.84, p < .001$) than did boys, there being no other significant univariate sex differences. The univariate School group effects are shown in Table 6.3. Despite ceiling effects, the high user group gave higher ratings of the addictiveness (but lower ratings of the lethality) of heroin. Among the other differences, the high user group rated tea, coffee, beer and spirits as more dangerous.

TABLE 6.3

Mean ratings of addictiveness and lethality of different substances: Low and High User Schools

	Addictiveness			*'Likely to kill'*		
School group	*Low*	*High*	*F*(1,722)	*Low*	*High*	*F*(1,722)
chocolate	2.79	3.12	3.03	1.55	1.69	.02
tranquillizers	5.32	5.73	5.05*	5.48	5.28	.26
tea/coffee	3.71	4.55	13.93***	2.06	2.35	7.38**
cigarettes	6.54	6.65	1.32	6.38	6.40	2.18
heroin	6.81	6.84	23.19***	6.97	6.90	6.07*
beer	5.72	5.78	1.58	5.15	5.23	5.11*
spirits	6.07	6.29	6.89**	5.70	5.99	5.04*
glue	6.57	6.59	.13	6.67	6.59	8.49**
cocaine	6.77	6.75	4.20*	6.94	6.82	.90
sleeping pills	5.40	5.59	6.22*	5.73	5.78	1.37
vitamin pills	3.99	4.07	11.25***	3.48	3.47	.04
LSD	6.21	6.32	.06	6.31	6.40	.30
cannabis	6.71	6.48	.23	6.73	6.42	2.54
N	474	352		188	538	

$*p < .05$ $\quad **p < .01$ $\quad ***p < .001$

(c) *Reasons why young people start taking drugs*

The multivariate effects for Sex ($F(20,726) = 2.68, p < .001$), School-group ($F(20,726) = 2.38, p < .001$), as well as the interaction ($F(20,726) = 1.61, p < .05$), achieved significance. Table 6.4 shows the means and univariate *F*s for the Sex and School group differences. As can be seen, girls were particularly more likely than boys to attribute drug use to problems at school and home, and to a wish to look grown up. Pupils in the high user schools were particularly more likely to make attributions to being given too much freedom, to boredom and to being in the wrong place at the wrong time.

TABLE 6.4

Mean ratings of reasons why young people start taking drugs.

	Sex			School group		
	Male	*Female*	*F*(1,745)	*Low*	*High*	*F*(1,745)
Parents	3.62	3.42	2.26	3.44	3.60	1.43
Something new	5.20	5.15	.16	5.16	5.20	.11
Don't think	5.25	5.45	2.28	5.31	5.38	.31
School problems	4.19	4.64	12.17***	4.30	4.53	3.15
Freedom	3.79	3.77	.03	3.54	4.02	9.28**
Pushed	3.03	6.26	4.89*	6.23	6.06	2.60
Home problems	4.84	5.18	7.61**	4.88	5.14	4.06
Right / wrong	4.07	4.05	.03	3.93	4.19	3.31
Bad company	5.93	6.14	3.85*	6.03	6.04	.01
Fun	5.60	5.74	1.34	5.61	5.74	1.13
Only once	6.20	6.26	.31	6.20	6.26	.29
Place / time	4.43	4.77	6.22*	4.42	4.78	6.62**
Feeling low	5.06	5.22	1.52	5.09	5.19	.59
Publicity	3.56	3.53	.03	3.59	3.51	.21
Bored	4.21	4.38	1.43	4.08	4.51	8.37**
Risks exciting	4.89	5.15	3.80	4.87	5.17	4.93**
Adult example	4.85	4.83	.03	4.96	4.72	2.47
Look grown up	5.41	5.76	7.10***	5.53	5.64	.74
Won't get a job	3.92	3.61	4.14*	5.68	5.85	1.29
Get hold easily	5.12	5.18	.19	5.09	5.21	.75
N	389	360		198	551	

$*p < .05$ $**p < .01$ $***p < .001$

(d) *Social competence*

This analysis revealed a significant Sex effect ($F(10, 780) = 7.90, p < .001$), the effect of School-group and the interaction being non-significant. Girls rated their social competence higher overall, especially in terms of understanding others' feelings (means: boys, 4.85, girls, 5.67; $F(1, 789) = 56.01, p < .001$), as well as getting on with teachers (means: 4.49, 4.96;

$F(1,789) = 13.03, p < .001$) and strangers (means: 4.71, 5.05; $F(1,789) = 8.02, p < .01$). They also rated as higher their ability to 'say no when you feel you shouldn't do something' (means: 5.56, 5.83; $F(1,789) = 4.83, p < .05$).

(e) *Beliefs about persuasion*

The multivariate effects of Sex ($F(10,771) = 4.21, p < .001$), School-group ($F(10,771) = 2.43, p < .01$) and the interaction ($F(10,771) = 2.08$, $p < .05$) were all significant. As may be seen in Table 6.5, five of the items showed significant Sex effects by univariate tests. In general, girls were more favourably disposed to methods consistent with a life-skills approach. The School- group effect was significant on just two items. The high user group was *more* in favour of a scare approach, and *less* in favour of helping young people to imagine themselves being offered heroin. Overall, giving as much information as possible was rated highest, and comparing tea and coffee with heroin was rated lowest.

TABLE 6.5

Mean ratings of persuasion methods.

	Sex			School group		
	Male	Female	$F(1,780)$	Low	High	$F(1,780)$
Scare	4.93	4.85	.25	4.87	5.11	7.85**
Alcohol/tobacco	4.35	4.55	1.59	4.38	4.53	.96
Tea/coffee	2.78	3.01	2.54	2.95	2.84	.55
Medicines	3.69	4.18	10.97***	4.00	3.86	.92
Imagine offer	4.92	5.37	9.18**	5.29	4.99	3.96*
Say no	5.70	6.03	6.76**	5.95	5.77	1.99
Talk about problems	5.55	6.10	23.07***	5.86	5.79	.32
Feel good	5.62	6.02	12.12***	5.90	5.73	2.11
Make decisions	5.69	6.03	10.06**	5.82	5.89	.39
Give information	6.33	6.37	.11	6.43	6.27	2.67
N	404	380		214	570	

$*p < .05$ $\quad **p < .01$ $\quad ***p < .001$

(f) *Most suitable person to teach about drugs*

There were no significant differences as a function of Sex, School-group, or their interaction. However, a test of the overall differences between the six target persons was highly significant ($F(5, 778) = 182.72, p < .001$). The targets were rated in the following ascending order of suitability: teacher (mean, 4.36), policeman (4.37), parent (4.44), nurse (5.41), doctor (5.89), ex-drug addict (6.40).

Discussion

The findings reported here should not be seen as any definitive statement on the *potential* effects that the "Double Take" package could have, were it to be thoroughly integrated into the school curriculum, and assigned sufficient time for class exercises and discussions. Unlike the study reported in chapter 5, the comparison of low and high user schools was strictly quasi-experimental, and should be viewed with all the caution that this term implies. Not only were the schools essentially self-selected, they also differed from each other on variables that could have influenced the dependent measures considered in the analyses.

Geographical area is one such factor, but although there were a variety of differences between schools, no consistent pattern of regional differences emerged. More importantly, perhaps, the low vs. high categorization was made on the basis of teachers' quantitative estimates of the use of "Double Take" in their schools, without regard to *how* the package was used, in which parts of the curriculum or in association with which other teaching materials or classes on drug-related topics. Unlike in the Chapter 5 study, we had no control over whether the emphasis was on "Minder" or "Thinking Twice". (In fact, it tended to be very much on "Minder", though some schools seemed to have shown "Thinking Twice" as well).

Predominantly, the package was used as part of the social or health education classes, although in one school it was used within religious education classes. Granted the relatively marginal status of such courses within the curriculum, and the consequential constraints in terms of class-hours available, it is not surprising that the amount of time given over to the use of the package was limited. On the other hand, the one school that (according to pupils) had used the package to a noticeable extent in the biology/science part of the curriculum produced the least impressive levels of pupil recall of lessons on specific topics related to drugs. This is not inconsistent with inferences drawn concerning the limited value of lessons about cigarette smoking when incorporated in biology/science as opposed to social education classes (Eiser, Morgan & Gammage, 1988).

Notwithstanding these difficulties, the analyses presented here show that greater use of "Double Take" was associated with a number of differences in pupils' attitudes and beliefs. These conclusions are broadly consistent across the two designs on which the analyses were based. Possibly the most encouraging result is that pupils from high user schools rated legal drugs (e.g. alcohol, caffeine, sleeping pills) as more dangerous generally than did those from low user schools. The ratings for heroin were so close to the extreme of the scale that the data should be interpreted cautiously, but even so there was a small but reliable increase in the perceived addictiveness of heroin, accompanied by a small decrease in its perceived lethality (when going from the low to the high user means). In terms of perceived reasons why young people take drugs, the main finding is that the high user pupils were more inclined than low user pupils to offer broadly situational explanations, such as 'being in the wrong place at the wrong time', together with other explanations including boredom, excitement, and 'too much freedom'. The results from the analyses of preferred methods of persuasion are somewhat disconcerting: high user pupils appeared to be (relative to low user pupils) not at all enthusiastic about 'decision-making' approaches, being significantly keener on a scare approach. Thus, even if their own attitudes had been changed by lessons incorporating more emphasis on decision skills (though we can be far from certain that the package was in fact generally used in such a way), this does not seem to have converted them to the educational philosophy which they themselves had experienced. Rather, these findings suggest that, in becoming more 'anti-drug' in certain respects, the high user pupils simply adopted a more punitive attitude towards the question of deterrence.

The data also show a number of trends across both low and high user schools. One with clear practical implications is that pupils regarded teachers, parents and police officers as least suitable informants about drug problems, but ex-drug addicts as the most suitable. Such responses should be seen as reflecting the fact that former drug-takers would be seen as 'knowing what they were talking about' rather than a comment on what particular message such informants might actually convey.

Last but not least, we found strong and consistent sex differences on many variables. It is apparent that girls were much more sympathetic to decision-making/life-skills approaches to drug education, were more likely to explain drug use in terms of personal problems, and rated their own social competence at relating to others more positively overall. One possible implication is that drug education might need to be slanted slightly differently for boys than for girls.

7

Attitudes, attributions and persuasion: How young people's ideas about drugs relate to their preferences for different strategies of prevention

Introduction

In the previous two chapters, we considered various differences between pupils' responses that were associated with different levels of use of "Double Take" in the respective schools. However, evaluation of the likely effectiveness of any such intervention should not simply depend on the detection of specific short-term effects, but should also include a consideration of how well matched the content of the intervention was to pupils' own views of drugs and drug-use. This is not to say that such views cannot themselves be influenced, but only that the initial acceptability of a particular approach to drug education may depend in part on its congruence with more general beliefs and values which pupils hold. In short, the impact of any message will depend on how well it is understood, and such understanding will depend on its relationship to prior knowledge and beliefs.

Thus, whereas the previous chapter considered differences between the schools, the present chapter compares individuals in terms of their differential acceptance of particular attitudes and beliefs. The latter include the questions relating to relationships with parents, dangerousness of different substances, social competence, explanations for why young people take drugs and ideas about the best way to prevent them doing so, and more general beliefs about the nature of drug-use and addiction.

The theoretical framework which guided the selection of questions and the analyses to be reported is eclectic. One central theme, however, is the notion that people's general attitudes and preferred courses of action are associated with why they believe particular events or conditions come about. This relates to social psychological research on attributions, or subjective explanations of events (see J.R. Eiser, 1986; Kelley & Michela, 1980). Applied to the present case, we can ask the question whether pupils' ideas about why young people take drugs can predict how they believe such behaviour can be best discouraged and prevented. Research in other contexts, such as with patients at drug-dependence clinics (Eiser & Gossop, 1979) and adult smokers (Eiser & van der Pligt, 1986) suggest that such beliefs may be important predictors of behaviour. Such an inquiry needs also to consider views held about the nature of drugs and their relative danger, the meaning of addiction, relationships with parents and general social competence. Such issues relate to the perceived context of adolescent drug-use, as well as to questions which the "Double Take" package was designed to raise.

Method

The data considered in this chapter were derived from all participants (i.e. all three conditions) of the experimental study described in Chapter 5, and from all participants (i.e. both age-groups) in the school comparison study described in Chapter 6. The total number of subjects was therefore 1,352, although this figure was reduced where some individuals failed to answer certain questions. Furthermore, one set of statements, ('Beliefs about drug-use') had been responded to only by those in the second sample. Otherwise, the following sets of questions, answered by both samples, were considered: perceptions of parental behaviour; dangerousness of different substances; reasons why young people start taking drugs; social competence; beliefs about persuasion.

Results

a) *Factor analyses*

We first conducted a series of principal components analyses, with varimax rotation, on each of the separate sets of statements, as described below.

(i) *Parental behaviour*

This analysis yielded two factors (with eigenvalues greater than 1.0). The first, accounting for 32.0% of the variance, we interpreted as a 'Protest' factor, in that it seemed to represent general complaints over the inconsistency or restrictiveness of parents' rules. The second factor, accounting for 15.8% of the variance, seemed to represent 'Autonomy', in other words, a perception by the respondents that they were not (or no longer) especially constrained in their behaviour by parental control or surveillance. Table 7.1 shows the factor loadings for these items.

TABLE 7.1

Principal components analysis of 'parental behaviour' items: Rotated factor matrix

	Factor 1 'Protest'	Factor 2 'Autonomy'
Item		
Parents change minds	.605	.283
Parents know where I am	.125	-.744
Decide for myself	.055	.623
Parents more strict than most	.716	-.171
Parents' rules don't make sense	.474	.495
Parents aren't interested	.366	.409
Parents treat me like a baby	.699	.083
Parents don't allow enough freedom	.780	.060
Eigenvalue	2.563	1.264

(ii) *Dangerousness of substances*

For purposes of this analysis, we summed the ratings of addictiveness and lethality to give an overall 'danger' score for each of the 13 substances. The factor analysis on these summed scores is summarized in Table 7.2. There were three factors, accounting respectively for 36.6%, 16.3% and 8.4% of the variance. The first was mainly an '*illicit drugs*' factor, comprising cocaine, heroin, solvent abuse, cannabis and LSD, but interestingly with moderately high loadings on cigarettes, sleeping pills and tranquillizers in addition. The second appears mainly a '*Food/medicine*' factor, including 'non-drugs' such as chocolate and vitamin pills, tea and coffee and prescribed drugs (tranquillizers and sleeping pills). The third was an '*Alcohol/tobacco*' factor.

TABLE 7.2

Principal components analysis of 'dangerousness' ratings: Rotated factor matrix

Item	Factor 1 'Illicit drugs'	Factor 2 'Food/medicine'	Factor 3 'Alc./tobacco'
Chocolate	-.158	.695	.112
Tranquillizers	.440	.486	.051
Tea/Coffee	-.091	.719	.173
Cigarettes	.526	.064	.553
Heroin	.798	-.115	.272
Beer/cider	.072	.237	.845
Spirits	.255	.233	.805
Glue/solvents	.794	.009	.280
Cocaine	.853	-.079	.231
Sleeping pills	.516	.558	.093
Vitamin pills	.116	.653	.120
LSD	.703	.157	.027
Cannabis	.737	.057	.010
Eigenvalue	4.755	2.115	1.096

(iii) *Reasons*

These 20 items yielded a more complex solution with five factors accounting respectively for 24.0%, 8.3%, 7.17%, 5.9% and 5.7% of the variance. The factor loadings are shown in Table 7.3. The first seemed to reflect '*Social pressure/ experimentation*'; the second, mainly '*Anticipation of adulthood*' (though with additional themes of risk-taking and availability); the third related to 'Mood'; the fourth to '*Problems/upbringing*'; and the fifth to

Table 7.3

Principal components analysis of 'reasons' items: Rotated factor matrix

Items	Factor 1 'Social pressure/ experimentation'	Factor 2 'Anticipation of adulthood'	Factor 3 'Mood'	Factor 4 'Problems/ upbringing'	Factor 5 'Situations/ morality'
Parents don't look after	.043	.119	−.051	.690	.077
Try new	.412	.243	.255	.128	−.044
Don't think	.507	.110	.026	.177	.054
Problems at school	.134	.036	.408	.630	−.073
Too much freedom	.161	.180	−.094	.516	.353
Pushed by peers	.605	.110	−.027	.176	−.014
Problems at home	.156	−.001	.362	.671	.020
No sense of right/wrong	.230	.109	−.136	.226	.698
Bad company	.714	.048	−.007	.097	.180
Fun	.654	.108	.301	−.076	.171
Will only be once	.686	.097	.170	−.019	.048
Wrong place/time	.285	−.022	.299	−.017	.613
Feeling low	.256	−.040	.691	.236	.150
Publicity	−.207	.298	.320	−.033	.543
Bored	.056	.311	.681	.075	.062
Risks exciting	.287	.476	.488	−.031	.069
Adults drinking/smoking	.058	.756	.049	.112	.127
Look grown up	.317	.711	−.005	.109	−.103
Won't get job	−.097	.452	.321	.161	.300
Get hold too easily	.204	.440	.142	.017	.144
Eigenvalue	4.805	1.653	1.427	1.181	1.131

'*Situations/ Morality*' (i.e. a combination of being in the wrong place, and having no sense of right or wrong).

(iv) *Social competence*

This analysis revealed three factors (see Table 7.4) accounting for 28.5%, 13.1% and 10.7% of the variance. The first seemed to reflect '*Social skills*', including dealings with peers, strangers, new places and understanding others' feelings. The second related clearly to 'Adults', and the third to 'Self-reliance'.

(v) *Beliefs about persuasion*

This analysis revealed two factors with eigenvalues above 1.0, and a third with an eigenvalue above 0.99. The three-factor solution appeared more useful on conceptual grounds, and is summarized in Table 7.5. The first factor (27.8% of the variance) involves endorsement of a '*Life-skills*' approach; the second (17.1% of the variance) reflects approval of discussion of '*Licit drugs*'; and the third (9.9% of the variance) is clearly a 'Scare' factor.

TABLE 7.4

Principal components analysis of 'social competence' items: Rotated factor matrix

	Factor 1 'Social skills'	Factor 2 'Adults'	Factor 3 'Self-relianace'
Item			
Peers	.515	.324	.026
Strangers	.842	-.010	.132
New places	.791	.020	.126
Adults	.363	.649	.084
Parents	-.068	.791	.109
Teachers	.122	.718	.105
Understand others	.434	.296	.185
Make decisions	.245	.027	.629
Say 'no'	-.045	.151	.775
Cheer up	.124	.089	.579
Eigenvalue	2.848	1.309	1.075

TABLE 7.5

Principal components analysis of 'persuasion' items: Rotated factor matrix

	Factor 1 'Life skills'	Factor 2 'Licit drugs'	Factor 3 'Scare'
Item			
Make really scared	.027	.051	.940
Discuss alcohol/tobacco	.112	.660	.292
Discuss tea/coffee	-.064	.755	-.080
Discuss medicines	.086	.830	-.026
Help imagine offer	.381	.370	.218
Help say no	.573	.107	.269
Help discuss problems	.735	-.006	-.027
Help feel good	.772	.003	.007
Help make decisions	.707	.018	-.039
Give information	.617	.117	.055
Eigenvalue	2.779	1.705	.993

(vi) *Beliefs about drug-use*

Four factors were revealed (see Table 7.6) accounting respectively for 17.9%, 15.9%, 11.9% and 10% of the variance. The first related to the perceived 'Benefits' of drug-use. The second was mainly a '*Positive prognosis*' factor, indicating that drug-users could give up and/or be treated, and were much like other people. The third seems closest to the 'Hooked' factor of the Eiser and Gossop (1979) and Eiser and van der Pligt (1986) studies, and it is interesting that the item about AIDS loads most heavily here (suggesting possibly a 'Junky' image of drug-takers). The fourth resembles the 'Sick' factor of the previous studies cited (but without confidence in the efficacy of medical help, which loads instead on Factor 2).

TABLE 7.6

Principal components analysis of 'drug-use beliefs' items: Rotated factor matrix

Item	Factor 1 'Benefits'	Factor 2 'Positive' prognosis'	Factor 3 'Hooked'	Factor 4 'Sick'
Terrified of withdrawal	.016	.058	.522	.196
Could give up	.015	.795	-.177	.074
Just like others	.323	.497	.251	-.088
More likely to get AIDS	.031	.129	.547	.371
Drug-addiction a sickness	-.083	.052	.201	.816
Drugs make you feel good	.701	.047	.177	-.295
Doctors can help	-.072	.702	.140	.060
Difficult to stop	-.004	-.039	.744	-.128
Can take for fun	.667	-.018	-.276	.389
Drugs relieve worries	.787	.025	.012	-.014
Eigenvalue	1.790	1.587	1.194	1.001

b) *Multiple regression analyses*

A series of multiple regression analyses were then conducted to see how well the respondents' scores on each of the three 'persuasion' factors could be predicted from their factor scores derived from the remaining analyses. Two analyses were conducted for each of the 'persuasion' factors. The first used the combined sample of subjects from the 'experimental' (Chapter 5) and 'regional' (Chapter 6) studies, with a total size of 1031 after exclusion of any with missing data, but did not include responses to the 'beliefs about drug-use' items. The second included this last category of items, but for this reason was performed on a restricted sample of 610, all from the 'regional' study. (However, the factor scores on the other sets of items were still calculated from the factor analyses performed on the combined sample.) Tables 7.7 and 7.8 show the results of these analyses for the larger and smaller samples respectively.

TABLE 7.7

Multiple regression analyses to predict each of the 'persuasion' factors from other factor scores (N = 1031). Beta weights where significance of t < .1

	Dependent	*variable*	
	Life-skills	Licit drugs	Scare
Predictors			
Protest			
Autonomy	−.083**		
Illicit drugs			
Food / medicine		.132***	
Alcohol / tobacco			−.086**
Social pressure	.232***		.159***
Antic. adulthood	.086**	.095**	
Mood	.183***		
Problems/upbringing	.057*	.053	
Situations/morality		.094**	.092**
Social skills	.197***		
Adults	.062	.064	
Self reliance	.089**		.073*
Multiple R	.448	.239	.241

$*p < .05$ $**p < .01$ $***p < .001$

The main findings were that endorsement of a 'Life-skills' approach to prevention related strongly to pupils' own social skills and self-reliance, and to attributions for drug-use particularly in terms of social pressure / experimentation and mood. Endorsement of discussion of 'Licit drugs' was most clearly linked to a greater belief in the dangers of 'food/ medicines' (with ratings of 'alcohol/tobacco' contributing comparatively little to the prediction) and also to explanations in terms of 'anticipation of adulthood' and 'situations/ morality'. Support for a 'Scare' approach related strongly to attributions to 'social pressure/experimentation' as well as to 'situations/morality'. The relative contribution of other predictors varies somewhat between the two analyses, but it appears that approval of a 'Scare' approach was also related to seeing illicit drugs as more dangerous but alcohol and tobacco as less so, and to greater confidence in one's 'self-reliance'.

TABLE 7.8

Multiple regression analyses to predict each of the 'persuasion' factors from other factor scores (N = 610). Beta weights where significance of t < .1

	Dependent	*variable*	
	Life-skills	Licit drugs	Scare
Predictors			
Protest	−.084*		
Autonomy			
Illicit drugs			0.86*
Food/medicine		.169***	.076
Alcohol/tobacco			−.069
Social pressure	.229***		
Antic. adulthood		.079	.123**
Mood	.169***		−.102*
Problems/upbringing	.091*		
Situations/morality		.070	.091*
Social skills	.207***		
Adults			
Self-reliance	.080*		.081*
Benefits	−.087*		
Positive prognosis	.103**		
Hooked	.128***		.080*
Sick			
Multiple R	.512	.235	.288

$*p < .05$ $**p < .01$ $***p < .001$

Although the responses to the 'beliefs about drug-use' items made some contribution to the prediction of the 'persuasion' factors, a rather clearer picture of the status of these beliefs comes from a second set of multiple regressions analyses (on the sample of 610) to predict each of the 'drug-use beliefs' factors from the remainder. These are shown in Table 7.9. Of especial interest is the finding that endorsement of a 'life-skills' approach contributed positively to the prediction of 'positive prognosis' and 'hooked' beliefs, but related negatively to beliefs in the 'benefits' of drug-use. Belief in such benefits was also related to explanations in terms of 'mood' but not in terms of social pressure or anticipation of adulthood.

TABLE 7.9

Multiple regression analyses to predict each of the 'beliefs about drug-use' factors from other factor scores (N = 610). Beta weights where significance of t < .1

	Dependent		*variable*	
	Benefits	Positive prognosis	Hooked	Sick
Predictors				
Protest			.071	
Autonomy	.089*			
Illicit drugs				
Food/medicine	.106*			
Alcohol/tobacco			.078	
Social pressure	−.121**			
Antic. adulthood	−.082*		.085	.079
Mood	.108**			
Problems/upbr.				
Situations/moral		.079		
Social skills	.108*			
Adults	−.102*			
Self-reliance				
Life-skills	−.094*	.127**	.154***	
Licit drugs				
Scare			.071	.083*
Multiple R	.359	.186	.304	.194

$*p < .05$ $**p < .01$ $***p < .001$

c) *Multivariate analyses of variance*

We next performed two multivariate analyses of variance, following the designs described in Chapter 6. The first was a 2 x 2 x 7 (Sex x Age-group x School) factorial design with the dependent variables being the factor scores from all the principal components analyses described above (i.e. including the 'drug-use beliefs' factors), but considering only the seven schools on which the 'regional' comparisons were based.

This analysis revealed significant multivariate effects for Sex ($F(20,547) = 2.46$, $p < .001$), Age-group ($F(20,547) = 4.33, p < .001$), School ($F(120, 3312) = 2.17$, $p < .001$) and Age-group x School ($F(120,3312) = 1.48, p < .001$), together with the three-way interaction ($F(120,3312) = 1.31, p < .05$). The low vs. high user contrast of the School effect ($F(20,547) = 2.81, p < .001$) and of the Age-Group x School interaction ($F(20,547) = 1.93, p < .01$) were significant.

Univariate tests (with *df* = 1,566) indicated that the Sex effect depended mainly on the following differences: compared with boys, girls saw themselves as having marginally less 'autonomy' from their parents ($F = 3.60, p < .1$), were more likely to favour explanations in terms of 'mood' ($F = 8.70, p < .01$) but less in terms of 'problems/upbringing' ($F = 5.75, p < .05$); they were also more likely to favour prevention strategies based on 'life-skills' ($F = 7.38, p < .01$) and discussion of 'licit drugs' ($F = 4.45, p < .05$), and less likely to regard drug-takers as 'sick' ($F = 9.22, p < .01$). Regarding the Age-group effect, older pupils gave higher ratings to their 'autonomy' from their parents ($F = 29.40, p < .001$), saw 'illicit drugs' ($F = 5.68, p < .05$) and, marginally, 'alcohol/tobacco' ($F = 2.86, p < .1$) as more dangerous. Comparatively speaking, the older pupils rejected explanations in terms of 'anticipation of adulthood' ($F = 6.60, p < .01$), 'problems/upbringing' ($F = 3.38, p < .1$) and 'situations/morality' ($F = 8.21, p < .01$), preferring to attribute drug-use to 'mood' ($F = 4.59, p < .05$). They also rated their interactions with 'adults' more negatively ($F = 10.75, p < .001$), and gave more optimistic ratings of the 'benefits' ($F = 9.18, p < .01$) of drug-use and of the 'positive prognosis' ($F = 6.17, p < .05$) for drug-takers.

With regard to the low vs. high user contrast, those in the low user school, comparatively speaking, rated their 'autonomy' from their parents as high ($F = 6.92, p < .01$), the danger of 'illicit drugs' ($F = 6.78, p < .01$), of 'food/medicine' ($F = 9.23, p < .01$) and, marginally, of 'alcohol/tobacco' ($F = 3.49, p < .1$) as low. They were less likely to explain drug-use in terms of 'situations/morality' ($F = 8.44, p < .01$) or, marginally, 'anticipation of adulthood' ($F = 3.48, p < .1$) or 'mood' ($F = 2.99, p < .1$). They were least keen on a 'scare' approach to prevention ($F = 6.68, p < .01$), and more optimistic about the 'positive prognosis' for drug-takers ($F = 3.93, p < .05$). The interaction between Age-group and the low vs. high user contrast depended on just one dependent variable: the tendency for 'illicit drugs' to be rated lower by the low user group was entirely dependent on the responses of the younger pupils ($F = 15.78, p < .001$).

The second analysis compared the high users with the larger group of low users, i.e. including the control group from the sample described in Chapter 5, but excluding the younger age-group from the later (Chapter 6) sample. This was a simple 2 x 2 (Sex x School-group) design, and yielded significant multivariate $Fs(16, 630)$ of 5.73, $p < .001$, for Sex, 2.30, $p < .01$ for School-group and 1.76, $p < .05$ for the interaction. Univariate tests ($df = 1, 645$) of the Sex effect suggested a few differences from the pattern of results in the previous analysis. Compared with boys, girls saw themselves as having less 'autonomy' from their parents ($F = 25.06, p < .001$), rated 'alcohol/tobacco' as less dangerous ($F = 13.86, p < .001$), and were more likely to attribute drug-use to 'social pressure/ experimentation' ($F = 4.54, p < .05$) and somewhat to 'mood' ($F = 2.88, p < .1$); they also gave higher evaluations of their own 'social skills' ($F = 9.53, p < .01$) and, marginally, of their interactions with 'adults' ($F = 3.54, p < .1$). In addition, girls were more likely to favour 'life-skills' approaches to prevention ($F = 13.43, p < .001$) and the discussion of 'licit drugs' ($F = 8.05, p < .01$). Equivalent tests of the School-group effect revealed that pupils from high user schools gave higher ratings of the danger of 'food/medicine' substances ($F = 8.92, p < .01$), but marginally lower ratings of the danger of 'illicit drugs' ($F = 3.55, p < .01$). The high user group were marginally more likely to favour explanations in terms of the 'situations/morality' factor ($F = 3.05, p < .1$), and were significantly keener on a 'scare' approach to persuasion ($F = 7.13, p < .01$). The significant interaction mainly depended on two items: the dangerousness of 'food/medicine', where the School-group effect was apparent only for females ($F = 6.73, p < .01$) and the 'mood' explanation factor, where the Sex factor occurred only in the high user group ($F = 6.81, p < .01$).

Discussion

Whereas there are many interrelationships among the variables which bear comment, the most interesting appear to be those between endorsement of different prevention strategies and other factors. The "Double Take" programme includes explicit emphasis on life-skills and decision-making, and "Thinking Twice" (though not "Minder") stresses continuities between licit and illicit drug-use. Although both parts of the package convey cautionary messages, neither represents a 'scare' approach. Despite this, as has been noted, those with greater exposure to the programme (mainly "Minder") declared themselves more in favour of a 'scare' approach, whereas 'life-skills' and discussion of 'licit drugs' was favoured more by girls than boys.

Greater acceptance of a 'life-skills' approach was related to pupils' own 'social skills' and 'self-reliance', suggesting a clear link between how these young people saw themselves and what they felt others might need to become so as to be less at risk with regard to taking up drugs. The association between acceptance of a 'life-skills' approach and a view of drug-use as arising from 'social pressure' and a desire for 'experimentation' (together with 'mood' causes) coincides closely with the philosophy upon which most life-skills programmes have themselves been based. However, a belief that 'social pressures' are important did not necessarily lead to preference for a 'life-skills' approach: this belief (together with a belief in the importance of 'situations/morality') contributed to the possibly more punitive attitude expressed by greater preference for a 'scare' approach. A concern with what we have termed 'anticipation of adulthood' (e.g. adult example, a wish to look grown up) combines with a belief in the continuities between more and less dangerous substances to predict favourable attitudes towards the strategy of talking about other substances (tea, coffee, alcohol, tobacco and medicines) at the same time as heroin.

The age-group differences suggest a shift from explanations in terms of 'extrinsic' to 'intrinsic' factors. In other words, the younger pupils were more likely than the older ones to attribute drug-use to 'anticipation of adulthood', 'problems/ upbringing' and 'situations/morality'. None of these factors deal directly with the possible effects of drugs *per se*. At the same time, the older pupils were the more likely to endorse 'mood' explanations and to assert that drugs might have 'benefits'. Thus, for the older age-group, there was relatively more of an emphasis on what drugs can do (in terms of controlling affective states, etc.), and less on what might be special about drug-takers and the circumstances in which they find themselves. This concern with control of affective states appears to have parallels with the development of attitudes towards cigarette smoking (J.R. Eiser, 1985; Eiser, Morgan & Gammage, in press; Marsh, 1984).

Finally, it is appropriate to consider the factor structure of the 'drug-use beliefs' items. These were partly based on items used in previous research with patients at a drug-dependence clinic (Eiser & Gossop, 1979) and adult smokers (Eiser & van der Pligt, 1986). In both these previous studies, a two-factor solution was favoured, with a distinction between being 'Hooked' (unable to give up) on the one hand, and 'Sick' on the other. It should be pointed out that these previous studies asked subjects to consider their own use of drugs or cigarettes, which did not apply here; the set of statements was by no means identical, and the smaller sample sizes (particularly in the Eiser & Gossop, 1979 study) means that any solution needed to be interpreted cautiously.

Even so, we might have expected, on the basis of these previous findings, that rejection of the 'benefits' items would combine with higher scores on the 'sick' factor, and that the 'positive prognosis' factor would subdivide, with the item asserting that doctors 'can help' loading positively on 'sick' and the belief that drug-takers can give up if they 'really wanted to' loading negatively on 'hooked'. Although some of the weaker loadings (see Table 7.6) are not entirely incompatible with these inferences, there are still important distinctions that would have been disguised by a two-factor solution. In particular, the special status of the 'benefits' factor appears particularly important. In that endorsement of this factor is greater among older pupils, but is negatively related to endorsement of a 'life-skills' approach, there would appear to be implications for educational interventions. Drug education, whether it incorporates 'life-skills' training or not, should provide full information about what drugs can do, and how they influence feelings and mood, for the worse as well as for the (short-term) better without overstressing the argument that young people only take drugs because other people influence them to do so. The intrinsic effects of drugs are dealt with in "Double Take", but this is perhaps a theme that deserves even more emphasis in the exercises, particularly those accompanying "Minder".

8

Analysis and synthesis: the status of "Double Take" in the school curriculum

Teachers' perceptions of the advantages of "Double Take"

Most teachers, including those who responded to the postal questionnaire described in chapter 2 and those we met in the process of collecting other data in schools, talked positively of the package. There is a considerable amount of material available to teachers organizing courses on drug abuse, and many used "Double Take" in combination with other material. The main advantages of "Double Take" are generally seen to be:-

1) The fact that it is freely distributed. While some Health Education Authorities and Institute for the Study of Drug Dependence leaflets are free (and their films can be freely obtained), other material using 'life-skills' approaches can be quite expensive. In some cases, schools which choose to use this material may be forced to accept sponsorship from local charities to fund the cost of buying books and training teachers. Many head-teachers are reluctant to accept charity money for material that is part of the curriculum. "Double Take" is clearly preferable to many for this reason.

2) Both videos, but particularly "Minder", are of a high technical quality. Pupils are used to seeing professional material everyday on television and in films, and are not tolerant of lower standards. While both "Minder" and "Thinking Twice" are acceptable in terms of quality of production, "Minder" is considerably more convincing in terms of the quality of the acting and credibility of the story-line. Teachers and pupils approve the quality of the acting and credibility of the story in "Minder"; they almost invariably criticize "Thinking Twice" on both counts.

3) The videos are accompanied by some fairly comprehensive teachers' notes and exercises for pupils. Many teachers have not attended relevant courses and are often not experienced with informal styles of teaching. In addition, social and health education courses are often taught by several teachers, some of whom are involved only on a temporary basis. Teachers' notes provide an essential function in guiding those who are new to drug education specifically and to more informal teaching methods in general.

Disadvantages and criticisms of the package

1) Many teachers like the package but do not feel that it is appropriate for their pupils. Their reasons are varied but include the fact that their pupils are too 'old', too 'young', too 'middle-class', too 'working-class', above or below average in intelligence. In addition, some teachers do not use the package because they do not feel that drug-taking is an issue for their pupils. It is also clear that, among teachers who do use the package, ratings of the package are affected by their own attitudes to drug-taking. Future attempts to promote this or similar packages should first address teacher attitudes to the issue. Many teachers need to be made aware that any pupil can become vulnerable in terms of drug-taking, not simply those conforming to their personal stereotype of a drug-addict. This applies especially to teachers in schools catering for predominantly middle-class children. While teachers do not all feel that illegal drugs are a problem for their pupils, they frequently acknowledge that alcohol is. They feel that health education should centre on alcohol, and tend to focus their teaching on alcohol in isolation from other drugs. This suggests that they need to be persuaded of the value of an approach, such as that taken in "Thinking Twice", that discusses continuities between legal and illegal drugs.

2) While the teachers' notes are welcome, they could undergo some revision. One of the main criticisms of the package is that it is time-consuming, and many teachers do not consider using "Double Take" for this reason. A shortened course would be invaluable. Teachers would like guidance as to how the package could be used where only one or two lessons are devoted to drug education. The notes could further be revised so as to suggest how "Double Take" can be integrated within existing courses or taught in conjunction with other material. Teachers would like guidance on how to tailor the course to their particular needs, particularly where limited time

is available for follow-up work. Some recommendations on which exercises to use or which points to emphasize would be helpful.

Factors limiting the success of the package

1) The first is concerned with teachers' ability and confidence to work with the package. Many teachers are involved on a temporary basis only, and have little formal knowledge of the topic or experience of the informal style of teaching required. In contrast to other issues where they are responsible for the organisation and content of their own lessons, in social and health education they are often given material by other teachers. In many cases, then, they are required to teach a course based on a package that they themselves have not selected and know little about. At the same time, they are not likely to have experience using the informal style of teaching in their original training course nor to have attended a relevant in-service course.

2) To a large extent, dissatisfaction is expressed with the organization and content of social and health education courses generally, rather than "Double Take" itself. While some schools do have well-structured courses covering a range of topics within these areas, other schools are still very much in the process of organisation and re-organisation. The task is far from simple. There is a wide range of topics which could be included in these courses (for example, smoking, alcohol, sex education, AIDS, child care and human development, finance and banking, vocational guidance, the law ...). There is only limited curriculum time available, and the courses are invariably seen as less important than traditional subjects. Some teachers, and pupils too, may well under-value health and social education courses, however much time and effort is put into them.

3) Inevitably, some of the pupils exercises are used more extensively than others. For "Minder", those involving character evaluations are seen to be helpful. Some of the more general exercises are difficult for younger or less able pupils. For example, sheet 8 (values) includes descriptions of some situations that pupils will not yet have encountered e.g., 'not declaring earnings in income tax returns is a justifiable way of making money.' Many of these items are complex and merit considerable discussion. Observations in schools suggests that the use of such an exercise often does not result in the balanced discussion that might be hoped. While pupils are able to

discuss an item such as 'it is OK to miss paying a bus or train fare if no-one asks for the money' and offer a range of explanations, the more complicated items simply result in endorsement of the socially accepted response - e.g. 'of course' it is not right to buy goods that you suspect have been obtained illegally.

While many of the exercises are commendable, they can be difficult to implement in a classroom setting. However good one's initial intentions, when dealing with a class of 30 or so pupils it is easy to revert to a traditional style of teaching. Organizing discussion or role-play activities for such a large number is very demanding for the teacher as well as resulting in intense noise levels! In addition, pupils themselves need to learn how to derive maximum benefit from a decision-making approach. Since pupils' previous experience is usually exclusively centred on traditional methods of teaching, they need to learn how to function in groups and participate in discussions.

Our data suggest that pupils are not always in favour of a life-skills or decision-making approach. Boys are considerably less enthusiastic than girls about strategies involving talking about personal feelings, and they give lower ratings of their own ability to empathize with others. Support for such an approach seems also to be linked to a view of adolescent drug-use as attributable to factors such as social pressures, a wish for experimentation and anticipation of adulthood. Belief in the importance of these factors seems rather distinct from a tendency to see drugs as useful in the short term as a way of controlling mood — yet we may speculate that a belief in the *benefits* of drug-use (stronger among older pupils) may constitute a significant incentive for those otherwise at risk.

Pupils generally approve of being given 'as much information as possible', but approval for a 'scare' approach too is far from negligible; curiously, it is stronger within those schools where the package (or at least "Minder") was more extensively used. The more damaging inference is that these pupils, having experienced a life-skills approach, were declaring that they might have preferred something else entirely. However, this may be to interpret their responses too literally. A less damaging interpretation is that (a) pupils did not fully recognize the (partial) life-skills approach they had experienced for what it was; and (b) in saying that they thought potential drug-takers should be made 'really scared'; they were mainly just expressing a more strongly negative attitude towards drug-use — something that might be regarded as an achievement of the programme. Even so, many pupils' reticence about the general approach needs to be acknowledged, and sympathetic teaching is essential to clarify the aims of the approach and to encourage the pupils' full participation.

Practical recommendations

While we acknowledge that these problems are unlikely to be easily overcome, it seems to us that the following may be helpful.

1) With regard to the fact that teachers are not always familiar with the topic or style of teaching, then good teacher support is critical. The role of Local Advisory Teachers for Drugs Education should not be overlooked. Many Advisory Teachers had not yet been in post for a full academic year, and their impact may still be limited. Certainly many schools involved in our evaluations had had no contact with Local Advisory Teachers. Their potential role in training teachers, either by organizing courses or visiting schools and helping to teach, should not be underestimated.

2) With regard to the fact that limited curriculum time is available for social and health education courses and that a large number of topics may be included, it is not necessarily helpful for teachers to be inundated with extensive courses for particular topics. However well-researched the content of the courses and however high the quality of the teaching materials, the package must still be integrated within the constraints of social and health education courses generally. Programme advisors need to acknowledge this. It is not always useful for a school to be confronted with a drugs education package that requires 5 hours of curriculum time, for example, if only a few more hours are available for the entire course.

It would be more helpful if it was emphasized that the package could be used effectively to teach pupils about issues other than drugs. "Double Take" could be used to introduce pupils to issues such as alcohol, smoking, criminality and the law and social relationships, as well as illicit drug-use. A more comprehensive approach to social and health education and acknowledgement of the constraints imposed on the curriculum in secondary schools might be helpful. Even so, there must be some acknowledgement that neither gains in knowledge nor changes in attitudes, let alone behaviour, are likely to be achieved without substantial commitment of curriculum time. As noted earlier, Connell *et al* (1985) reported that 40-50 hours of curriculum time were necessary to produce *stable* effects on attitudes and behaviour. Using a related 'social skills' approach to the prevention of alcohol problems among U.S. Marines, Cameron (personal communication) reports that a programme extending over 45 hours is thought desirable.

Comparing and contrasting "Minder" and "Thinking Twice"

In the teachers' notes accompanying "Thinking Twice" (p.34) it is pointed out that "Thinking Twice" has two goals: - to teach decision-making skills and knowledge of drugs. The notes go on to describe the programme as being 'anti-experimentation' in orientation, and suggest that a further approach in terms of preventing casualties among experimenters may be needed in addition. Two options are considered available to teachers wishing to provide this further education; the use of the manual "Health Careers" or the "Minder" video and exercises. While it would be very convenient to conclude that "Thinking Twice" and "Minder" constituted two contrasting but complementary approaches to drug education which could be used together to provide a balanced programme satisfying both these aims, we have some reservations about such a recommendation.

In that each video seems, on the basis of these results, to have been successful with regard to particular implicit aims, we do not see it as our role to identify which was 'better'. Such a judgement could only be made on the basis of a choice between the aims themselves, and these, in turn, seem to reflect broader ideological conceptions of what health education in general should try to achieve. If the aims of the package are attitude and behaviour change, then "Minder" seems clearly the more persuasive. Although it is beyond the scope of a study such as this to determine whether any attitude changes would be translated into greater behavioural rejection of drug-use, "Minder" seems to use many classic persuasive techniques and to use them well. Although quite 'informative' at the level or portraying circumstances and some consequences of drug-use, it is unambiguous in its prescriptive message — heroin is unquestionably bad, and anyone who starts using it can easily become addicted.

A quite different view of health education is that its purpose should always be informative, and never prescriptive. According to this view, the success of health education is to be viewed in terms of how well-informed the target group becomes with regard to the issue in question, even if no demonstrable behaviour change results. The goal is therefore that people should be able to make more 'informed choices' for themselves, whatever these choices might be. Thus, 'Thinking Twice' continually emphasises that young people have to make decisions about drugs for themselves. The difficulty that then arises, however, is one of determining what kind of information is going to be most relevant to young people in their earliest encounters with illicit drug-use. Knowing that tea and coffee, say, also contain a 'drug' might well lead to an underestimation of the more specific dangers of heroin use. On the other hand, more differentiated information about how and why 'drugs' vary in addictiveness and lethality could well act as a deterrent to experimentation with more harmful drugs, whether legal or illegal. Information of the latter kind, however, may be more difficult to convey. The point of this that is a different selection of information can have different behavioural implications. Hence, any intervention that leaves its target audience partially informed (even if better informed than before) may (unintentionally) be prescriptive in its implications.

Much therefore depends on whether the aim of the package is to be regarded as primarily persuasive or educational, and if educational, whether its focus should be on 'drugs' as a general category or dangerous drug-use in particular. Here the aims and interests of the 'consumers' of the package, as well as of its sponsors and producers, require consideration.

One of the difficulties in developing a school-based drugs education curriculum may be that, while there are some similarities in reasons why pupils take legal and illegal drugs, and some similarities between the aims of prevention programmes, there are also critical differences. Pupils may begin to smoke, drink alcohol or take illegal drugs because of peer pressure, because they have poorly developed self-esteem or because they lack assertiveness. Their reasons may also relate to the climate within their families or because they perceive themselves to be doing badly academically. They may smoke or take drugs for some of these or many other reasons, but it may not be possible to identify specific reasons for any individual. Programmes that do not take account of such a range of precipitating factors affecting drug-use are less likely to be successful.

By the same token, the aims of programmes concerned with preventing alcohol or cigarette use need not be the same as those concerned with prevention of illicit drug taking. Educators may simply wish to promote abstinence, or delay onset of use. More complex goals may involve teaching responsible use or informed decision making. For example, educators may accept that pupils will drink alcohol, and restrict their goal to teaching pupils about the dangers of irresponsible or excessive drinking (e.g. drunk driving). Alternatively, educators may wish to replace 'unhealthy' behaviours such as smoking or drinking with more desirable behaviours, such as increasing exercise or improving diet. From this perspective, drugs education is a highly complex issue, and one that may well merit higher status in the school curriculum. Similar conclusions should perhaps be made about the life-skills approach in itself. The traditional view of education, and the one that is probably held by the majority of teachers and parents, is that schools should teach pupils facts, while various social and life-skills are acquired through a process of trial and error. Yet increasingly, such skills are seen not only to be mediating variables in behaviours such as drug-use, but also a means of enhancing overall functioning (Meichenbaum *et al*, 1981). The impact of "Double Take" is determined as much by teachers' beliefs about the value of drug education in particular and life-skills training in general, as by any technical limitations of the package itself.

Appendix A

Questionnaires used by teachers

Name of person completing questionnaire:

Position in school:

Information about the school

Name:

Address:

Postcode:

Size (please state approximate number of pupils):

Type (please tick appropriately)

☐ Independent ☐ Maintained

☐ Selective ☐ Comprehensive

☐ Single-sex boys ☐ Single-sex girls ☐ Boys and girls

Age range of pupils

☐ 10-13 ☐ 11-16 ☐ 11-18 ☐ 12-16 ☐ 12-18 ☐ 13-18 ☐ 16-18

How many *full time* teachers are employed?

What is the *teacher-pupil* ratio?

Approximately what percentage of pupils receive free school meals?

1 a) *When was 'Double Take' received by the school?*

Approximate date:

1 b) Is there still a copy in the school? ☐ Yes ☐ No

2 a) *How was the decision to order 'Double Take' made?* (please tick any that apply)

☐ In a staff meeting

☐ By memo

☐ Individual discussions

2 b) How many teachers in the school were involved in the decision to order 'Double Take'?

2 c) How many teachers have seen 'Double Take'?

2 d) Have parents had the opportunity to see 'Double Take'?

2 e) Have any sessions on drug education been organised for parents at the school? (please tick appropriately)

☐ More than one session ☐ One session ☐ None

3) *Drug education in school*

Please estimate the *average* number of curriculum hours during (a) 1985-6; (b) 1986-7, devoted or, to be devoted firstly to drug education *in genral*, and secondly to the use of 'Double Take' (and the exercises based on it) for each age group.

a) *1985-6 academic year*

Drug education	☐ 11-12	☐ 12-13	☐ 13-14	☐ 14-15	☐ 15-16
'Double Take'	☐ 11-12	☐ 12-13	☐ 13-14	☐ 14-15	☐ 15-16

b) *1986-7 academic year*

Drug education	☐ 11-12	☐ 12-13	☐ 13-14	☐ 14-15	☐ 15-16
'Double Take'	☐ 11-12	☐ 12-13	☐ 13-14	☐ 14-15	☐ 15-16

c) In which parts of the curriculum has it generally been decided to use 'Double Take'? (please tick any that apply)

☐ Spare periods arising from staff absence, etc.
☐ Social education/Tutor groups/Design for living
☐ Health education
☐ English
☐ Biology/other sciences
☐ Other (please specify)

d) About how many teachers in your school do you think use 'Double Take' (or parts of it) regularly?

e) Are other people (apart from teachers) involved in drug education in your school on a regular basis?

- ☐ School nurse/doctor
- ☐ LEA drug adviser
- ☐ Health education officer
- ☐ Other (please specify)

f) To your knowledge is 'Double Take' *generally* being used:

- ☐ with relatively equal emphasis on both parts ("Minder" and "Thinking Twice")
- ☐ with more emphasis on "Minder"
- ☐ with more emphasis on "Thinking Twice"
- ☐ with considerable differences in emphasis between individual teachers

g) Have teachers followed the exercises suggested in the Teachers' Notes?

Accompanying "Minder":

☐ Not at all ☐ Selectively ☐ Closely

Accompanying "Thinking Twice"

☐ Not at all ☐ Selectively ☐ Closely

h) How would you personally rate the "Double Take" package?

	very unhelpful						very helpful
As a whole	☐	☐	☐	☐	☐	☐	☐
The "Minder" video	☐	☐	☐	☐	☐	☐	☐
The "Thinking Twice" video	☐	☐	☐	☐	☐	☐	☐
The exercises/Teachers' Notes for "Minder"	☐	☐	☐	☐	☐	☐	☐
The exercises/Teachers' Notes for "Thinking Twice"	☐	☐	☐	☐	☐	☐	☐

i) Have teachers designed their own exercises to accompany:

"Minder" : ☐ yes ☐ No

"Thinking Twice": ☐ yes ☐ No

j) Do you use any other drug education programmes? ☐ Yes ☐ No

If yes, please give details:

Which of these, if any, do you consider preferable to 'Double Take'?

Why?

k) Have you (or any other teacher at your school, to your knowledge) attended any of the following?

- ☐ TACADE course on drug education
- ☐ TACADE course on "Double Take"
- ☐ LEA drug adviser course on drug education
- ☐ Other (please specify)

l) *If you found that a pupil was experimenting with drugs, what would you do?* (please tick whichever apply)

- ☐ Inform a parent
- ☐ Inform the family doctor
- ☐ Inform the police
- ☐ Contact LEA drug adviser
- ☐ Counsel pupil yourself
- ☐ Contact school counsellor
- ☐ Other (please specify)
- ☐ Inform school nurse/doctor
- ☐ Inform LEA
- ☐ Inform EWO
- ☐ Suspend the pupil
- ☐ Discuss drugs with all pupils
- ☐ Discuss drugs with all parents
- ☐ Introduce a drug education programme

m) Does the school or LEA have any policy on dealing with children known to be experimenting with drugs?

4 *Do you believe that, in general, young people start taking drugs like heroin because:*

	definitely no						definitely yes
They find it exciting to take risks.	☐	☐	☐	☐	☐	☐	☐
They're having a problem at school.	☐	☐	☐	☐	☐	☐	☐

There's too much publicity about drugs.	☐	☐	☐	☐	☐	☐	☐
They're having problems at home.	☐	☐	☐	☐	☐	☐	☐
They see adults drinking and smoking.	☐	☐	☐	☐	☐	☐	☐
They think it will be fun.	☐	☐	☐	☐	☐	☐	☐
Their parents don't look after them properly.	☐	☐	☐	☐	☐	☐	☐
They're feeling low at the time.	☐	☐	☐	☐	☐	☐	☐
They get into bad company.	☐	☐	☐	☐	☐	☐	☐
They don't think about the consequences.	☐	☐	☐	☐	☐	☐	☐
They're pushed into it by other young people.	☐	☐	☐	☐	☐	☐	☐
They want to look grown up.	☐	☐	☐	☐	☐	☐	☐
They want to try something new.	☐	☐	☐	☐	☐	☐	☐
They're given too much freedom.	☐	☐	☐	☐	☐	☐	☐
They've no sense of right and wrong.	☐	☐	☐	☐	☐	☐	☐
They tell themselves it will only be once.	☐	☐	☐	☐	☐	☐	☐
They're bored.	☐	☐	☐	☐	☐	☐	☐
They feel they won't get a job.	☐	☐	☐	☐	☐	☐	☐
They can get hold of drugs too easily.	☐	☐	☐	☐	☐	☐	☐
They don't know enough about what drugs can do	☐	☐	☐	☐	☐	☐	☐

5 *Do you believe that, in order to persuade young people not to try drugs like heroin, it is a good idea to:*

	definitely no						definitely yes
Make them really scared.	☐	☐	☐	☐	☐	☐	☐
Talk about alcohol and tobacco at the same time as heroin	☐	☐	☐	☐	☐	☐	☐
Talk about tea and coffee at at the same time as heroin	☐	☐	☐	☐	☐	☐	☐
Talk about medicines at the same time as heroin	☐	☐	☐	☐	☐	☐	☐
Help them to imagine being offered heroin	☐	☐	☐	☐	☐	☐	☐
Involve their parents in drug education	☐	☐	☐	☐	☐	☐	☐

Help them to practice saying no	☐	☐	☐	☐	☐	☐	☐
Help them to talk about personal problems and worries	☐	☐	☐	☐	☐	☐	☐
Help them to feel good about themselves	☐	☐	☐	☐	☐	☐	☐
Help them to make decisions for themselves	☐	☐	☐	☐	☐	☐	☐
Help them to imagine what it would be like to be offered heroin	☐	☐	☐	☐	☐	☐	☐

6) Do you have any other general comments about "Double Take"?

7) *Next year we would like to evaluate pupils' reactions to "Double Take" in a small number of schools. Would you be willing for some of the pupils to be involved in this research?*

☐ Yes definitely ☐ Yes possibly ☐ No

Appendix B

Questionnaires used by pupils

The sections on pages 1 to 6 were used in questionnaires in all schools.

The sections on page 7 were used only in the study described in chapter 5.

The sections on pages 8 and 9 were used only in the study described in chapter 6.

This questionnaire is to find out what you know and think about drugs and people who take them. There are no right or wrong answers to the questions, so just write down what **you** think. We will not show your questionnaire to any teachers or parents. Please answer all the questions. Thank you for filling in the form.

Name:

I am ______________ years old

I am a boy / girl (please circle one)

Class (tutor's name) ____________________________

Please read the following statements carefully and tick (√) the box which best describes you. Please tick one box only.

I have never smoked a cigarette, not even a puff	
I have only tried smoking once or twice	
I used to smoke sometimes, but I now don't	
I smoke sometimes but don't smoke as much as one cigarette a week	
I usually smoke between one and six cigarettes a week	
I usually smoke between six and twenty cigarettes a week	
I usually smoke more than twenty cigarettes a week	

	Yes	No	I don't smoke
Do you usually smoke every day?	☐	☐	☐

How do you think you are doing in your school work?

	Not at all well						Very well indeed
Please tick one box	☐	☐	☐	☐	☐	☐	☐

Do you ever drink alcohol?

	Yes	No
Alone	☐	☐
Only with boys	☐	☐
Only with girls	☐	☐
With both girls and boys	☐	☐
With parents	☐	☐

Have you ever got really drunk?

	Never	Only once	More than once
Please tick one box	☐	☐	☐

How true is each of the following statements for you?

	Almost always true	Often true	Sometimes true	Rarely true	Never true
My parents keep changing their minds about what I can and cannot do.	☐	☐	☐	☐	☐
My parents always know where I am and what I 'm doing.	☐	☐	☐	☐	☐
My parents are more strict than most parents.	☐	☐	☐	☐	☐
My parents' rules don't make much sense.	☐	☐	☐	☐	☐
My parents aren't interested in my problems and the decisions I have to make.	☐	☐	☐	☐	☐
My parents still treat me like a baby.	☐	☐	☐	☐	☐
My parents do not allow me enough freedom to do what I want.	☐	☐	☐	☐	☐

Do you think that there is much risk of people becoming addicted to any of these?

	definitely no						definitely yes
Chocolate	☐	☐	☐	☐	☐	☐	☐
Tranquillizers	☐	☐	☐	☐	☐	☐	☐
Tea or coffee	☐	☐	☐	☐	☐	☐	☐
Cigarettes	☐	☐	☐	☐	☐	☐	☐
Heroin	☐	☐	☐	☐	☐	☐	☐
Spirits (whisky, gin, vodka, etc.)	☐	☐	☐	☐	☐	☐	☐
Glue/solvent sniffing	☐	☐	☐	☐	☐	☐	☐
Cocaine	☐	☐	☐	☐	☐	☐	☐
Sleeping pills	☐	☐	☐	☐	☐	☐	☐
Vitamin pills	☐	☐	☐	☐	☐	☐	☐
LSD	☐	☐	☐	☐	☐	☐	☐
Cannabis (pot,dope, etc.)	☐	☐	☐	☐	☐	☐	☐

Do you think that there is much risk of people being killed by any of these?

	definitely no						definitely yes
Chocolate	☐	☐	☐	☐	☐	☐	☐
Tranquillizers	☐	☐	☐	☐	☐	☐	☐
Tea or coffee	☐	☐	☐	☐	☐	☐	☐
Cigarettes	☐	☐	☐	☐	☐	☐	☐
Heroin	☐	☐	☐	☐	☐	☐	☐
Spirits (whisky, gin, vodka, etc.)	☐	☐	☐	☐	☐	☐	☐
Glue/solvent sniffing	☐	☐	☐	☐	☐	☐	☐
Cocaine	☐	☐	☐	☐	☐	☐	☐
Sleeping pills	☐	☐	☐	☐	☐	☐	☐
Vitamin pills	☐	☐	☐	☐	☐	☐	☐
LSD	☐	☐	☐	☐	☐	☐	☐
Cannabis (pot,dope, etc.)	☐	☐	☐	☐	☐	☐	☐

Why do young people start taking drugs? Is it because: -

	definitely no						definitely yes
Their parents don't look after them properly.	☐	☐	☐	☐	☐	☐	☐
They want to try something new.	☐	☐	☐	☐	☐	☐	☐
They don't think about the consequences.	☐	☐	☐	☐	☐	☐	☐
They're having a problem at school.	☐	☐	☐	☐	☐	☐	☐
They're given too much freedom.	☐	☐	☐	☐	☐	☐	☐
They're pushed into it by other young people.	☐	☐	☐	☐	☐	☐	☐
They're having problems at home.	☐	☐	☐	☐	☐	☐	☐
They've no sense of right and wrong.	☐	☐	☐	☐	☐	☐	☐
They get into bad company.	☐	☐	☐	☐	☐	☐	☐
They think it will be fun.	☐	☐	☐	☐	☐	☐	☐
They tell themselves it will only be once.	☐	☐	☐	☐	☐	☐	☐
They're in the wrong place at the wrong time.	☐	☐	☐	☐	☐	☐	☐
They're feeling low at the time.	☐	☐	☐	☐	☐	☐	☐
There's too much publicity about drugs.	☐	☐	☐	☐	☐	☐	☐
They're bored.	☐	☐	☐	☐	☐	☐	☐
They find it exciting to take risks.	☐	☐	☐	☐	☐	☐	☐
They see adults drinking and smoking.	☐	☐	☐	☐	☐	☐	☐
They want to look grown up.	☐	☐	☐	☐	☐	☐	☐
They feel they won't get a job.	☐	☐	☐	☐	☐	☐	☐
They can get hold of drugs too easily.	☐	☐	☐	☐	☐	☐	☐

How much, on average, do you spend on yourself each week?

None	50p	£1	£1.50	£2.00	£2.50	£3.00	£4.00	£5.00	+£5-10	Over £10
☐	☐	☐	☐	☐	☐	☐	☐	☐	☐	☐

How well do you generally: -

	not at all well						very well indeed
Get on with people of your own age.	☐	☐	☐	☐	☐	☐	☐
Get on when you meet people you don't know	☐	☐	☐	☐	☐	☐	☐
Get on when you go to new places.	☐	☐	☐	☐	☐	☐	☐
Get on with adults.	☐	☐	☐	☐	☐	☐	☐
Get on with your parents	☐	☐	☐	☐	☐	☐	☐
Get on with your teachers.	☐	☐	☐	☐	☐	☐	☐
Understand other people's feelings.	☐	☐	☐	☐	☐	☐	☐
Make decisions for yourself.	☐	☐	☐	☐	☐	☐	☐
Say 'no' when you feel you shouldn't do something.	☐	☐	☐	☐	☐	☐	☐
Cheer yourself up when you feel low.	☐	☐	☐	☐	☐	☐	☐

Do you think that in order to persuade young people not to try drugs like heroin, it is a good idea to:

	definitely no						definitely yes
Make them really scared.	☐	☐	☐	☐	☐	☐	☐
Talk about alcohol and tobacco at the same time as heroin	☐	☐	☐	☐	☐	☐	☐
Talk about medicines at the same time as heroin	☐	☐	☐	☐	☐	☐	☐
Help them to imagine being offered heroin	☐	☐	☐	☐	☐	☐	☐
Help them to practice saying no	☐	☐	☐	☐	☐	☐	☐
Help them to talk about personal problems and worries	☐	☐	☐	☐	☐	☐	☐
Help them to feel good about themselves	☐	☐	☐	☐	☐	☐	☐
Help them to make decisions for themselves	☐	☐	☐	☐	☐	☐	☐
Give them as much information as possible	☐	☐	☐	☐	☐	☐	☐

Of the following people, who do you think is the most suitable to teach young people about the problem of taking drugs?

	definitely no						definitely yes
Parent	☐	☐	☐	☐	☐	☐	☐
Ex-drug addict	☐	☐	☐	☐	☐	☐	☐
Teacher	☐	☐	☐	☐	☐	☐	☐
Policeman	☐	☐	☐	☐	☐	☐	☐
Doctor	☐	☐	☐	☐	☐	☐	☐
Nurse	☐	☐	☐	☐	☐	☐	☐

What is a '*stimulant*'?

Write down the names of as many '*stimulant*' drugs as you can.

Applied to drug taking, what does '*tolerance*' mean?

What is meant by *addiction*?

Why is it more dangerous to take drugs when you 've been drinking alcohol?

Why is it more dangerous to inject drugs than take them by mouth?

Name the part of the body that is most at risk if you take drugs:

Why do you think the part of the body you have just named is more at risk than any other?

What is a 'Class A' drug?

Why do you think it is difficult to stop taking a drug like heroin?

Write as many reasons as you can think of why it's a good idea not to start taking drugs.

Can you name the drug or group of drugs which is:

a) Responsible for killing the greatest number of young people?

b) Was given to pilots during the 2nd World War to help them stay awake all night?

c) Is given to mums having babies?

d) Used to be used as an anesthetic?

e) Is used in the treatment of rheumatism and arthritis?

f) Is used in the treatment of diabetes?

g) Used to be used as a slimming pill?

What is a downer?

Write down the names of as many 'downer' drugs as you can.

Since September
do you remember *any* lessons about the following drugs or things to do with drug-taking?

	Yes	No
Heroin	☐	☐
Glue/solvent sniffing	☐	☐
Cannabis (pot etc.)	☐	☐
Cigarettes	☐	☐
Alcohol	☐	☐
Cocaine	☐	☐
Any other drug	☐	☐
Drug taking and AIDS	☐	☐
Advertising of cigarettes and/or alcohol	☐	☐

How much do you agree with the following statements:-

	Strongly disagree			undecided			Strongly agree
Drug-takers are terrified of withdrawal	☐	☐	☐	☐	☐	☐	☐
If drug-takers really wanted to they could give up drugs	☐	☐	☐	☐	☐	☐	☐
Drug takers are just like other people in lots of ways	☐	☐	☐	☐	☐	☐	☐
Drug-takers are more likely to get AIDS	☐	☐	☐	☐	☐	☐	☐
I think of drug-addiction as a sickness	☐	☐	☐	☐	☐	☐	☐
Drugs can really make you feel good	☐	☐	☐	☐	☐	☐	☐
I'm sure that doctors can help drug takers give up drugs	☐	☐	☐	☐	☐	☐	☐
Once you start taking drugs, it's very difficult to stop	☐	☐	☐	☐	☐	☐	☐
You can take drugs for fun without getting hooked	☐	☐	☐	☐	☐	☐	☐
Drugs can really make you less worried and anxious	☐	☐	☐	☐	☐	☐	☐

Here is a list of films about drugs and drug taking. Please tick any that you remember seeing.

Gail is dead.

Minder

Chase the bandwagon

It's your life

Free to choose

Better dead

Just say no

Grange Hill

BBC 'Drugwatch'

Thinking Twice

Drugs and Nervous System

Since September:

About *how many* lessons do you remember having about drugs and drug-taking in each of the following classes.

	No Lessons	1-3 Lessons	4-9 Lessons	10 or more Lessons
...in biology/science classes	☐	☐	☐	☐
...in health/social education classes	☐	☐	☐	☐
...in tutor groups	☐	☐	☐	☐
...in religious education classes	☐	☐	☐	☐
...in other classes	☐	☐	☐	☐

(Please say what these were ...)

References

Adelson, R. & Goldfried, M. (1970) Modeling and the fearful child patient. *Journal of Dentistry for Children, 37*, 476-489.

Alexander, C.N. Jr. & Campbell, E.Q. (1968) Balance forces and environmental effects: Factors influencing the cohesiveness of adolescent drinking groups. *Social Forces, 46*, 367-374.

Argyris, C. (1968) Conditions for competence acquisition and theory. *Journal of Applied Behavioral Science, 4*, 147-177.

Arkin, R., Roemhild, H., Johnson, C., Luepker, R. & Murray, D. (1981) The Minnesota Smoking Prevention Program: A seventh-grade health curriculum supplement. *Journal of School Health, 51*, 611-616.

Armstrong, R.W., Rosenbaum, P.L. & King, S.M. (1987) A randomized controlled trial of a 'buddy' programme to improve children's attitudes toward the disabled. *Developmental Medicine and Child Neurology, 29*, 327-336.

Bandura, A. (1977) *Social Learning Theory.* Englewood Cliffs, New Jersey: Prentice Hall.

Battjes, R.J. & Bell, C.S. (1985) Future directions in drug abuse prevention research. In C.S. Bell & R. Battjes (Eds.) *Prevention research: Deterring drug abuse among children and adolescents.* NIDA Research Monograph 63. A RAUS Review Report. DHHS.

Bauman, K.E. (1980) *Preventing adolescent drug use: The utility structure and marijuana.* New York, Praeger.

Blum, R., Garfield, E., Johnstone, J. & Magistad, J. (1978) Drug education: Further results and recommendations. *Journal of Drug Issues, 8*, 379-426.

Botvin, G.J. (1983) Prevention of adolescent substance abuse through the development of personal and social competence. In Glynn, T. & Leukeveld, C. (Eds.) *Preventing Adolescent Drug Abuse: Intervention Strategies.* DHHS Publication No (ADM) 83-128. Washington D.C. U.S. Government Printing Office.

Botvin, G.J. & Eng, A. (1982) The efficacy of a multicomponent approach to the prevention of cigarette smoking. *Preventive Medicine, 11*, 199-211.

Botvin, G.J. & Wills, T.A. (1985) Personal and social skills training: Cognitive–behavioral approaches to substance abuse prevention. In Bell, C.S. & Battjes, R. (Eds.) *Prevention research: Deterring drug abuse among children and adolescents.* National Institute on Drug Abuse Research Monograph 63. DHSS publication no. (AOM) 85-1334. Washington, D.C. Superintendent of Documents, U.S. Government Printing Office. Pp. 8-49.

Bruhn, J., Philips, B. & Gouin, H. (1975) The effects of drug education courses on attitudinal change in adult participants. *International Journal of Addictions, 10*, 65-96.

Burstein, S. & Meichenbaum, D. (1979) The work of worrying in children undergoing surgery. *Journal of Abnormal Child Psychology, 7*, 121-132.

Chen, T.T.C. & Winder, A.E. (1983) Teacher's perceptions related to smoking education between 1973 and 1982. *Journal of Drug Education, 15*, 125-138.

Cleary, P.D., Hitchcock, J.L., Semmer, N., Flinchbaugh, L.J. & Pinney, J.M. (1986) *Adolescent smoking: Research and health policy.* Discussion paper.

Connell, D.B., Turner, R.R., & Mason, E.F. (1985) Summary of findings of the School Health Education Evaluation: Health promotion effectiveness, implementation and costs. *Journal of School Health, 55*, 316-321.

DHSS, Treatment and rehabilitation. Report of the Advisory Council on the Misuse of Drugs, HMSO 1982.

Dupont, R.L. (1987) Prevention of adolescent chemical dependency. In *Pediatric Clinics of North America, 34*, 495-506.

Durell, J. & Bukoski, (1984) Preventing substance abuse: The state of the art. *Public Health Reports, 99*, 25-31.

Eiser, C. & Town, C. (1987) Teachers' concerns about chronically sick children: Implications for paediatricians. *Developmental Medicine and Child Neurology, 29*,

Eiser, J.R. (1985) Smoking: The social learning of an addiction. *Journal of Social and Clinical Psychology, 3*, 446-457.

Eiser, J.R. (1986) *Social psychology: Attitudes, cognition and social behaviour.* Cambridge: Cambridge University Press.

Eiser, J.R. & Gossop, M.R. (1979) "Hooked" or "sick": Addicts' perceptions of their addiction. *Addictive Behaviours, 4*, 189-191.

Eiser, J.R. & van der Pligt, J. (1986) Smoking cessation and smokers' perceptions of their addiction. *Journal of Social and Clinical Psychology, 4*, 60-70.

Eiser, J.R., Morgan, M. & Gammage, P. (1988) Social education is good for health. *Educational Research, 30, 1*, 20 - 25.

Eiser, J.R., Morgan, M. & Gammage, P. (submitted) Belief correlates of perceived addiction in young smokers.

Evans, R.I. (1976) Smoking in children: Developing a social psychological strategy of deterrence. *Preventive Medicine, 5*, 122-127.

Evans, R.I., Rozelle, R.M., Maxwell, S.E., Raines, B.E., Dill, C.A., Guthrie, P.C., Henderson, A.H. & Hill, P.C. (1981) Social modeling films to deter smoking in adolescents. Results of a three-year field investigation. *Journal of Applied Psychology, 66*, 399-414.

Festinger, C. (1957) *A Theory of Cognitive Dissonance*, Evanston, Illinois: Row, Peterson.

Flay, B.R. (1985) What we know about the social influences approach to smoking prevention: Review and recommendations. In C.S. Bell & R. Battjes (Eds.) *Prevention research: Deterring drug abuse among children and adolescents.* NIDA Research. Monograph 63. A RAUS Review Report. DHSS.

Flay, B., d'Avernas, J., Best, J., Kersell, M. & Ryan, K. (1983) Cigarette smoking: Why young people do it and ways of preventing it. In P. McGrath & P. Firestone (Eds.) *Pediatric and Adolescent Behavioral Medicine*, New York: Springer-Verlag.

Goldstein, A.P., Sherman, M., Gershaw, N.J., Sprafkin, R.P., & Glick, B. (1978) Training aggressive adolescents in prosocial behavior. *Journal of Youth & Adolescence*, *1*, 73-92.

Goodstadt, M.S. (1978) Alcohol and drug education models and outcomes. *Health Education Monographs*, *6*, 263-279.

Hackler, J.C. (1978) *The Prevention of Youthful Crime: The Great Stumble Forward.* Toronto, Methuen Press.

Halleck, S. (1970) The great drug education hoax. *The Progressive*, *34*, 1-7.

Halliday, G.W. (1976) Effect of fact valence on drug attitude. *Journal of Drug Education*, *6*, 89-95.

Higgins, C.W., Dunn, J.D. & Warmack, D. (1983) Comparisons of attitudes of smoking and non-smoking teachers toward smoking education in schools and the health consequences of smoking. *Health Education*, 24-27, Jan/Feb.

Hindmarsh, I. (1972) The pattern of drug abuse among school children. *Bulletin of Narcotics*, *24*, 23-26.

Home Office Report, 1986. Tackling drug misuse: A summary of the government's strategy.

Horan, J.J. (1972) An improved scale for quantifying drug abuse behavior. *Unpublished Research Instrument.* The Pennsylvania State University.

Horan, J.J. & Harrison, R.P. (1981) Drug Abuse. In B.B. Lahey & A.E. Kazdin (Eds.) *Advances in Clinical Child Psychology Volume 4*, New York: Plenum Press. Pp.283-330.

Horan, J.J., Westcott, T.B., Vetovich, C. & Swisher, J.D. (1974) Drug usage: An experimental comparison of three assessment conditions. *Psychological Reports*, *35*, 211-215.

Hurd, P., Johnson, C., Pechacek, T., Bast, C., Jacobs, D. & Luepker, R. (1980) Prevention of cigarette smoking in seventh grade students. *Journal of Behavioral Medicine, 3*, 15-28.

Janiver, R.L., Guthmann, D.R. & Catalano, R.F. Jnr. (1980) Reports of the National Juvenile Justice Assessment Centers: An Assessment of Evaluation of Drug Abuse Prevention Programs. Washington, D.C., U.S. Government Printing Office.

Jessor, R. (1982) Problem behavior and developmental transition in adolescence. *Journal of School Health*, 295-300.

Jessor, R., Collins, M.I. & Jessor, S.L. (1972) On becoming a drinker: Social-psychological aspects of an adolescent transition. In F.A. Seixas (Ed.) *Nature and Nurture in Alcoholism.* New York: Annals of the New York Academy of Sciences. Pp. 199-213.

Johnston, L.D., O'Malley, P.M. & Bachman, J.G. (1986) Drug use among American highschool students, college students and other young adults: National trends through 1985. Rockville, M.D. National Institute on Drug Abuse. DHHS Oub. No (ADM) 86-1450. Washington D.C.

Kandel, D. (1978) Homophily, selection and socialization in adolescent friendships. *American Journal of Sociology, 84*, 427-436.

Kandel, D.B. & Logan, J.A. (1984) Patterns of drug use from adolescence to young adulthood: 1. Periods of risk for initiation, continued use and discontinuation. *American Journal of Public Health, 74*, 660-666.

Kelley, H.H. & Michela, J.L. (1980) Attribution theory and research. *Annual Review of Psychology, 31*, 457-501.

Kinder, B.N., Pape, N.E. & Walfish, S. (1980) Drug and alcohol education programs: A review of outcome studies. *The International Journal of the Addictions, 15*, 1035-1054.

Kinsey, B.A., Nash, J. & Dodson, N. (1975) A comparative study of nonopiate clinical patients: Implications for education and prevention. *Journal of Drug Education, 5*, 141-150.

Leventhal, H. & Cleary, P.C. (1980) The smoking problem: A review of the research and theory in behavioral risk modification. *Psychological Bulletin*, *88*, 370-405.

Leventhal, H., Safer, M.A. & Panagis, D.M. (1983) The impact of communications on the self-regulation of health beliefs, decisions and behaviors. *Health Education Quarterly*, *10*, 3-28.

Luepker, R.V. Johnson, C.A., Murray, D.M. & Pechacek, T.F. (1983) Prevention of cigarette smoking - three year follow-up of an evaluation program for youth. *Journal of Behavioral Medicine*, *6*, 53-62.

MacDonald, D.I. (1987) Patterns of alcohol and drug use among adolescents. In *Pediatric Clinics of North America*, *34*, 275-288.

Machen, J.B. & Johnson, R. (1974) Desensitization, model learning, and the dental behavior of children. *Journal of Dental Research*, *53*, 83-90.

Maddox, G. & McCall, B.C. (1964) *Drinking among teenagers*, New Brunswick, N. Jersey, Rutgers Center of Alcohol Studies.

Marsh, A. (1984) Smoking: Habit or choice? *Population Trends* (HMSO), *36*, 14-20.

Mason, M.L. (1973) Drug education effects. *Dissertation Abstracts*, *34*, (4-B). 418.

Mathews, W.M. (1975) A critique of traditional drug education programs. *Journal of Drug Education*, *5*, 57-64.

McAlister, A., Perry, C., Killen, J., Slinkard, L. & Maccoby, N. (1980) Pilot study of smoking, alcohol and drug abuse prevention. *American Journal of Public Health*, *70*, 719-721.

McGuire, W.J. (1964) Inducing resistence to persuasion. In Berkowitz, L. (Ed.) *Advances in Experimental Social Psychology*, (Vol.1) New York, Academic Press.

Meichenbaum, D.H. (1971) Examination of model characteristics in reducing avoidance behavior. *Journal of Personality and Social Psychology*, *17*, 298-207.

Meichenbaum, D.H., Butler, L. & Gurson, L. (1981) Toward a conceptual model of social competence. In J.D. Wine & M.D. Smye (Eds.) *Social Competence*, New York: Guildford Press.

Melamed, B.G. & Siegel, L.J. (1975) Reduction of anxiety in children facing hospitalization and surgery by use of filmed modeling. *Journal of Consulting and Clinical Psychology, 43*, 511-521.

Michela, J.L. & Contento, I.R. (1984) Spontaneous classification of foods by elementary school aged children. *Health Education Quarterly, 11*, 57-76.

Milgram, G. (1976) A historical review of alcohol education research and comments. *Journal of Alcohol and Drug Education*, 2:2, 1-16.

Morgan, H.G. & Hayward, A. (1976) The effects of drug talks to school children. *British Journal of the Addictions, 71*, 285-288.

Moskowitz, J., Schaps. E. & Malvin, J. (1982) Process and outcome evaluation in primary prevention: The Magic Circle program. *Evaluation Review, 6* 775-788.

Parker, J., Pool, Y., Rawle, R. & Gay, M. (1986) *Problem drug use in Bristol. The final report of the Avon Drug Abuse Monitoring Project.* Unpublished report to the DHSS.

Pentz, M.A. (1980) Assertion training and trainer effects on unassertive and aggressive adolescents. *Journal of Counselling Psychology, 27*, 76-83.

Perry, C., Killen. J., Slinkard, L. & McAlister, A. (1980) Peer teaching and smoking prevention among junior high school students. *Adolescence, 15*, 277-281.

Perry, D., Maccoby, N. & McAlister, A. (1980) Adolescent smoking prevention: a third year follow-up. *World Smoking Health, 5*, 41-45.

Petchers, M.K. & Singer, M.I. (1987) Perceived benefit of drinking scales. Approach to screening for adolescent alcohol abuse. *Journal of Pediatrics, 110*, 977-984.

Peterson, L. & Ridley-Johnson, R. (1984) Pediatric hospital response to survey of pre-hospital preparation for children. *Journal of Pediatric Psychology, 5*, 1-7.

Robins, L.N. & Przybeck, T.R. (1985) Age of onset of drug use as a factor in drug and other disorders. In C.J. Jones & R.J. Battjes (Eds.) *Etiology of drug abuse: Implications for prevention.* National Institute on Drug Abuse Research Monograph 56. DHSS Publication No. (ADM) 85-1335. Washington, D.C. Superintendent of Documents, U.S. Government Printing Office.

Rosenblitt, D.L. & Nagey, D.A. (1973) The use of medical manpower in a seventh grade drug education program. *Journal of Drug Education, 3*(1), 39-56.

Saslawsky, D.a. & Wertele, S.K. (1986) Educating children about sexual abuse: Implications for pediatric intervention and possible prevention. *Journal of Pediatric Psychology, 11*, 235-246.

Schaps, E. Bartolo, R. D., Moskovitz, J., Palley, C. S. & Churgin, S. (1981) A review of 127 drug abuse prevention program evaluations. *Journal of Drug Issues, 11*, 17-43.

Schaps, E., Churgin, S., Palley, C.S., Takata, B., & Cohen, A.Y.C. (1980) Primary prevention research: A preliminary review of program outcome studies. *The International Journal of the Addictions*, 15:5, 657-676.

Schlegel, R.P. & Norris, J.E. (1980) Effects of attitude change on behavior for highly involving issues: The case of marijuana smoking. Addictive Behaviors, *5*, 113-124.

Schinke, S.P. (1981) Interpersonal skills training with adolescents. In M. Hersen, R.M. Eisler & P.M. Miller (Eds.) *Progress in Behavior Modification* Vol. II. New York: Academic Press.

Smart, R. & Fejer, D. (1974) The effects of high and low fear messages about drugs. *Journal of Drug Education, 4*, 225-235.

Smith, B.C. (1973) Values clarification in drug education: A comparative study. *Journal of Drug Education, 3*, 369-376.

Smith, P.B. & Gorry, G.A. (1980) Evaluating sex education programs. *Journal of Sex Education and Therapy, 6*, 17-23.

Staulcup, H., Kenward, K. & Frigo, D. (1979) A review of federal primary alcoholism efforts. *Journal of Studies in Alcohol, 40*, 943-968.

Stuart, R.B. (1974) Teaching facts about drugs: Pushing or preventing? *Journal of Educational Psychology, 66*, 189-201.

Stuart, R.B. & Schuman, M.C. (1972) Tripping and toking in mid-America: A survey of teenage drug abuse in four Michigan communities. Lowing, Mich: Office of Drug Abuse and Alcoholism,

Swift, B., Dorn, N. & Thompson, A. (1974) *Evaluation of drug education*, London. ISDD.

Swisher, J.D. (1976) Mental Health: The care of preventive health education. *Journal of School Health, 46*, 386-391.

Swisher, J.D., Crawford, J., Goldstein, R. & Yura, M. (1971) Drug education: Pushing or preventing? *Peabody Journal of Education, 49*, 68-75.

Swisher, J.D. & Horan, J.J. (1973) The Pennsylvania State University Drug Education Evaluation Scales, Part I: Drug Attitude Scale. In A. Abrams, E. Garfield & J.D. Swisher (Eds,) *Accountability in Drug Education: A model for evaluation*, Washington D.C., Drug Abuse Council.

Thompson, E.I. (1978) Smoking education programs, 1960-76. *American Journal of Public Health, 68*, 250-257.

U.S. Public Health Service (1979) *Smoking and health: A Report of the Surgeon General* Department of Health, Education and Welfare, U.S. Public Health Service Publication No.79-50066) Washington D.C., U.S. Government Printing Office.

Vernon, D.T.A. & Bailey, W.C. (1974) The use of motion pictures in the psychological preparation of children for induction of anesthesia. *Anesthesiology, 40*, 68-74.

Warner, R.W., Swisher, J.D. & Horan, J.J. (1973) Drug abuse prevention: A behavioral approach. National Association of Secondary School Principals Bulletin, *57*, 49-54.

Wiener, R.S.P. (1970) *Drugs and school children.* London, Longmans.

Weisheit, R.A. (1983) The social context of alcohol and drug education implications for program evaluations. *Journal of Alcohol and Drug Education*, *29*, 72-81.

Westervelt, V.D., Brantley, J. & Ware, W. (1983) Changing children's attitudes toward physically handicapped peers: Effects of a film and teacher-led discussion. *Journal of Pediatric Psychology*, *8*, 327-344.

Wright, J.D. & Pearl, L. (1981) Knowledge and experience of young people regarding drug abuse between 1969 and 1979. *British Medical Journal*, *282*, 793-796.

Yamaguchi, K. & Kandel, D.B. (1984) *Patterns of drug use from adolescence to young adulthood: II. Sequences of progression. American Journal of Public Health*, *74*, 668-672.

Zachary, R.A., Friedlander, S., Huang, L.N., Silverstein, S. & Leggott, P. (1985) Effects of stress-relevant and -irrelevant filmed modeling on children's responses to dental treatment. *Journal of Pediatric Psychology*, *10*, 383-402.